Steve Blackman

Understanding Ourselves

Contents

YOUR BODY	Your amazing body machine	2
	Building blocks of life	4
	Staying alive	6
	Every breath you take	8
	Eating to live	10
	Waste disposal	12
	Blood of life	14
	The body's pump	16
	Keeping control	18
	Your framework of bones	20
	Every move you make	22
YOUR SENSES	Look and listen	24
	Smells good, tastes good	26
	Skin deep	28
KEEPING HEALTHY	What you eat	30
	Enough to eat	32
	Keeping clean	34
	Exercise and resting	36
	Germs	38
	Medicines and drugs	40
GENETICS	What you look like	42
	It runs in the family	44
GROWING UP	Growing up, growing older	46
	Index	48

Cover photograph:
Swimming is a very good way of helping to keep fit.

Coordinating author:
Terry Jennings

Language consultant:
Diana Bentley

Additional contributions:
Nick Axten, Claire Axten

Note: Some spreads have been specially prepared for easier access. These are identified in **bold** print in the Contents' list above.

YOUR BODY

Your amazing body machine

Your body is like an amazing machine made up of **many different parts**, all joined together. Some parts are on the outside and can be easily seen. Many parts are on the inside. The inside parts are just as important, even though you cannot see them.

How you look

Even though everyone has a slightly different appearance (*even identical twins*), all bodies are basically the same. For example, we all have arms, legs, and a head. All of these parts join onto the part called the trunk.

The appearance of your body depends on your skeleton, your muscles, your skin, your age, and whether you are male or female. For example: tall people have larger skeletons; athletes can build up large and powerful muscles; older people may have wrinkled skin.

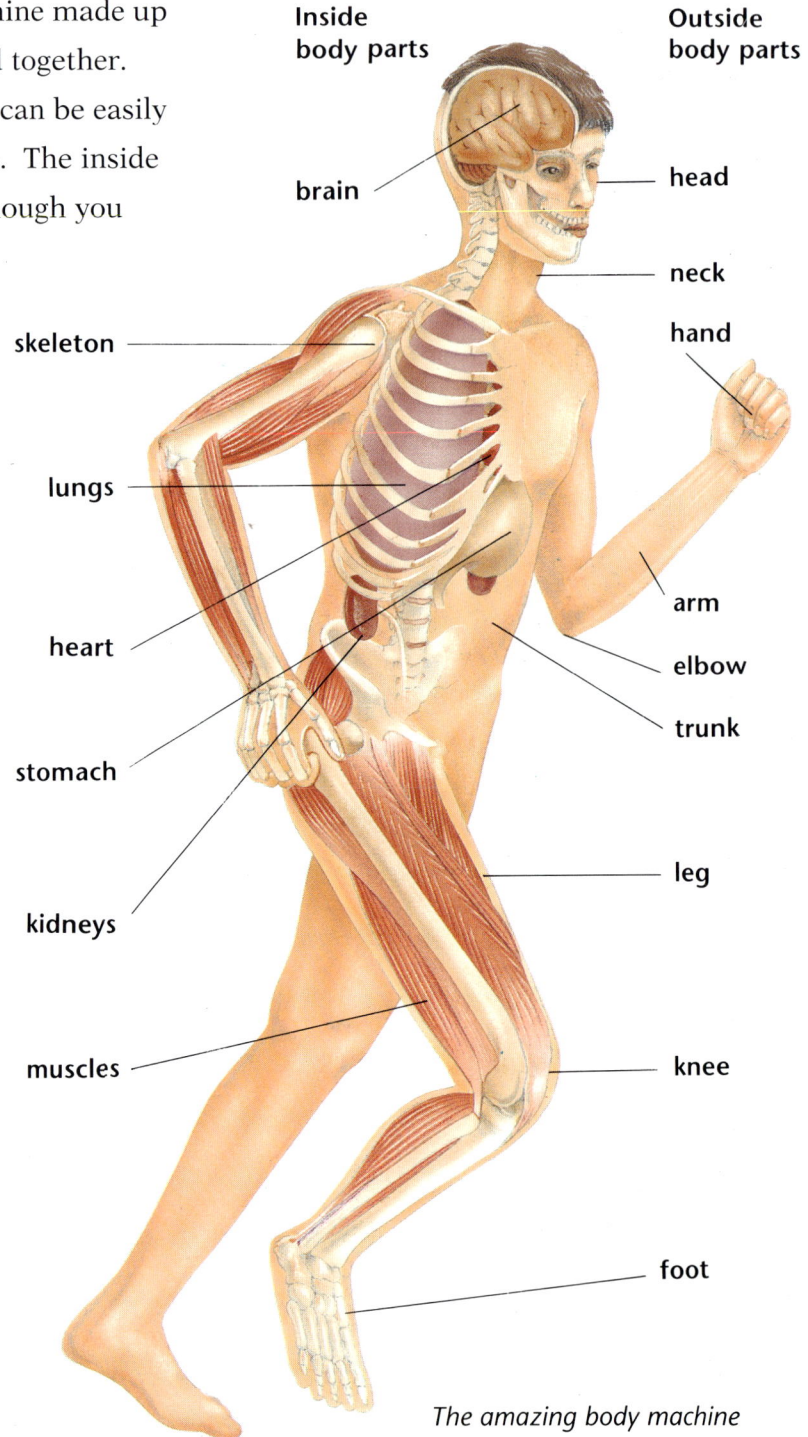

Inside body parts: brain, skeleton, lungs, heart, stomach, kidneys, muscles

Outside body parts: head, neck, hand, arm, elbow, trunk, leg, knee, foot

The amazing body machine

2

You and your friends

You could be the same age as your friend, but you could be a different height. One of you might be thinner than the other. Your eyes, hair, and skin could be different to those of your friend. All of these differences are important. They are some of the things that make you a **unique individual**.

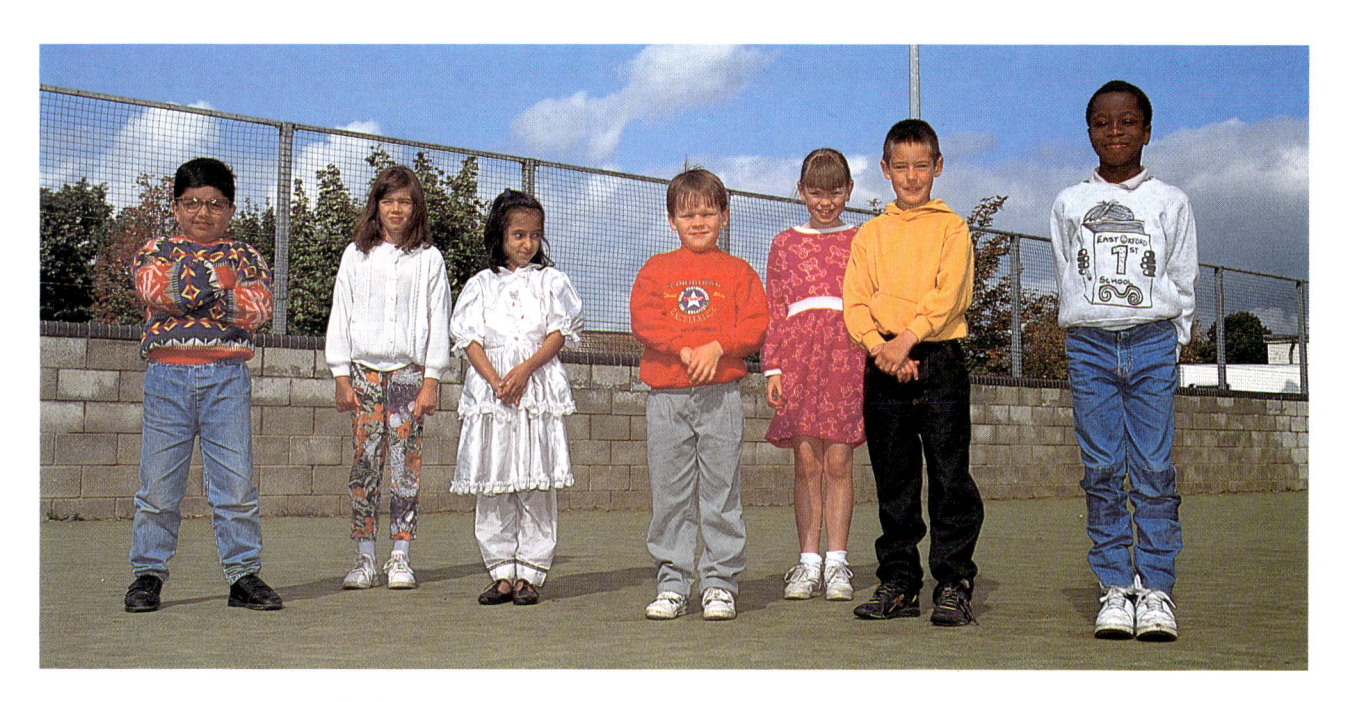

Everyone is a unique individual.

Keeping you alive

Every day your body has many different things to do to keep you alive and healthy:

- you breathe
- you eat and drink
- your heart beats
- you exercise
- you pass waste
- you rest and relax
- you sleep

🍎 Did you know that your body is mostly made up of water? Nearly three-quarters of your body weight is water.

🍎 **Focus**

many different parts

unique individual

YOUR BODY

Building blocks of life

Everyone is made up of millions of tiny building blocks called **cells**. Cells are the building blocks of life. Every part of your body is made up of different kinds of cells. Each kind of cell has a special job to do. It is no good trying to look for your cells. They are far too tiny to be seen without using a microscope.

🍎 **Human beings begin life as a *single* cell.**

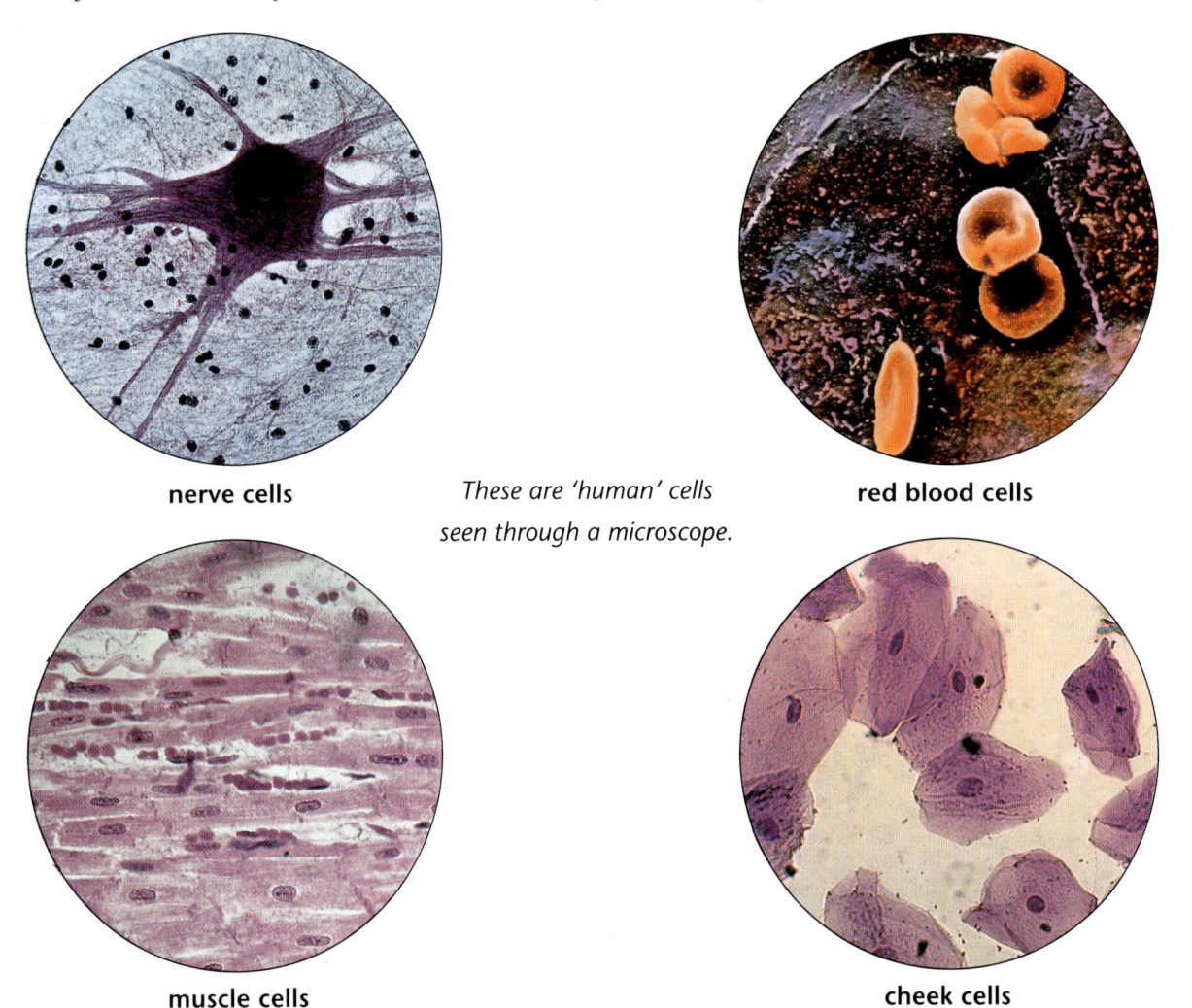

nerve cells

These are 'human' cells seen through a microscope.

red blood cells

muscle cells

cheek cells

Shapes of cells

The cells in your body are different shapes and sizes. Some are flat, others are round, and some are even square shaped.

4

The make up of a cell

Despite being different shapes, most cells have the same basic parts. The main centre part of a cell is called the **nucleus**. The nucleus controls the cell. It keeps the cell working on its own **special job**.

How a cell works

You already know that everyday your body takes in food, breathes, and gets rid of waste. Did you know that every tiny cell in your body is doing exactly the same? Every single cell takes in food, breathes, and gets rid of waste.

How cells grow

Some of your cells grow in size, that is they get bigger. Other cells grow in number, that is more of them are made. We say they **multiply**. Cells multiply by splitting into two equal parts, each with its own nucleus.

🍎 **There are thought to be about 50 thousand million cells in the body of an adult human.**

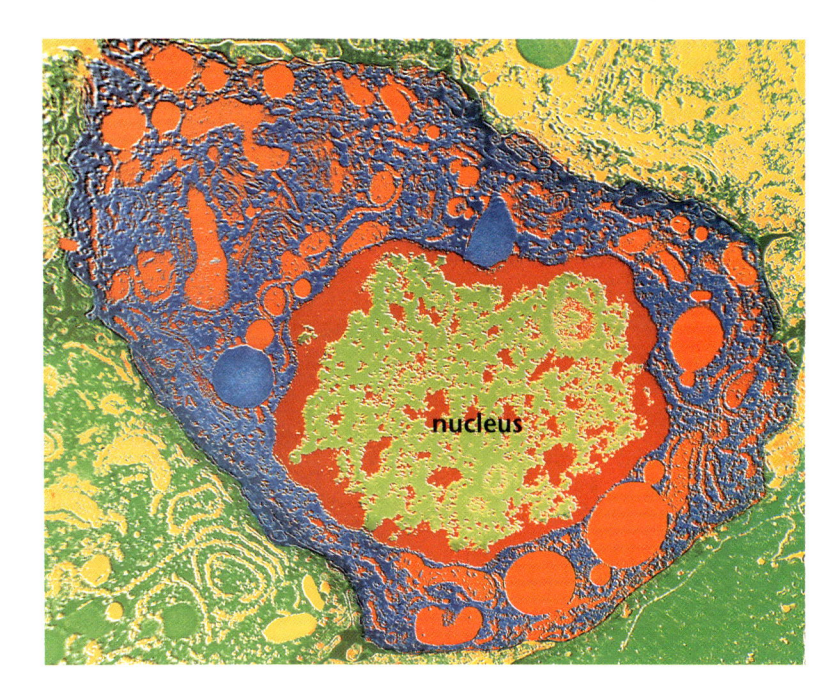

The make up of a cell (about 10,000 times larger than life: the colours are false)

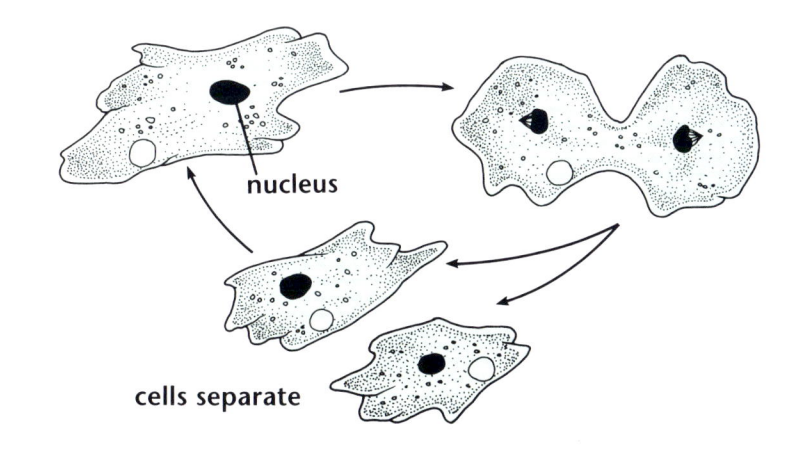

Some cells grow in number by splitting.

🍎 **Focus**　　cell　　nucleus　　special job　　multiply

YOUR BODY

Staying alive

Cells that do the same job are usually grouped together. These groups of cells are called **organs**. Each organ has its own position in your body, and its own job.

Some organs in your body are essential for staying alive. Without a brain, or a heart, or lungs you would die. Some of your organs help you to live, but are not essential to life. You could continue to live without your eyes or ears.

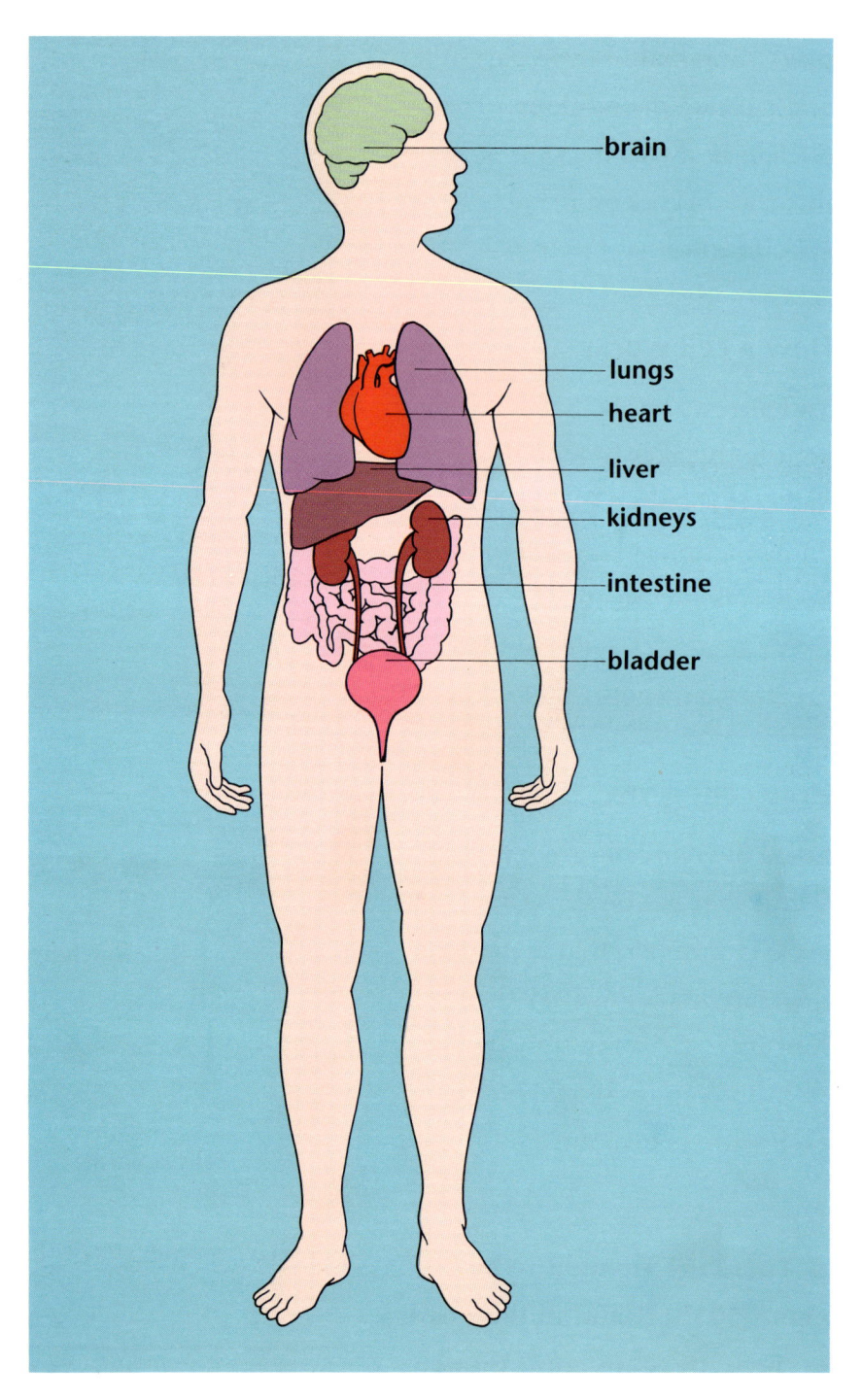

Some organs of your body

6

The stomach

Your stomach helps to digest food you have eaten. When food is digested it provides energy to your body cells. Sometimes you can feel your stomach mixing and churning the food as it is being digested.

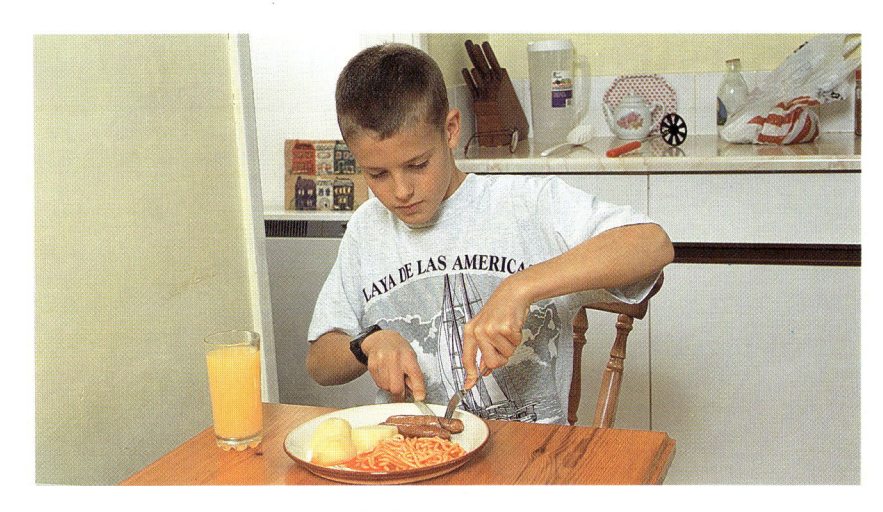

The food you eat is only partly digested in your stomach.

The lungs

You have two lungs inside your chest. As you breathe, your chest expands and your lungs take in air. When you breathe out, you empty your lungs of this air.

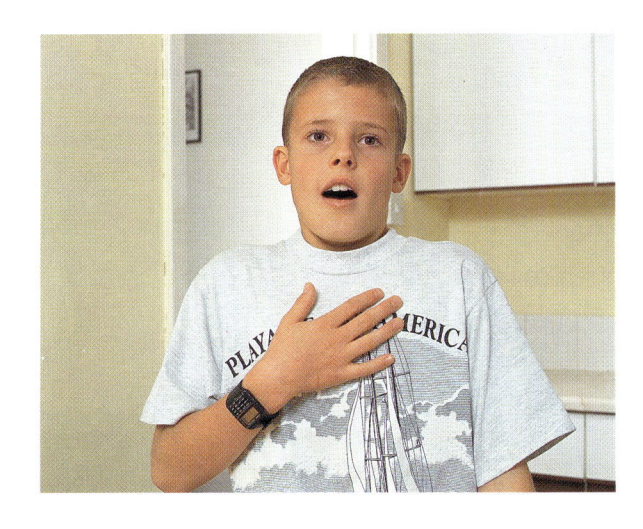

You can feel your chest expand when you take a deep breath.

The heart

Your heart is a very powerful muscle that works all the time. It never rests. It pumps blood around to every part of your body. When you exercise, your heart pumps faster.

🍎 **An elephant's heart beats about 25 times each minute. A mouse's heart beats about 500 times each minute. Your heart beats about 90 times each minute.**

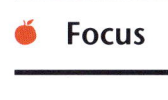

🍎 **Focus**

organ

YOUR BODY

Every breath you take

When you **breathe** in, you are supplying your body with fresh **oxygen**. When you breathe out you are getting rid of air and **carbon dioxide** which your body cannot use.

Bodies need oxygen

We all need oxygen to stay alive. Oxygen helps to give us energy to move about and grow. Oxygen passes through thin walls in your **lungs** and into your **blood**. Your blood carries the oxygen to all parts of your body. Carbon dioxide is passed from the blood back through the thin lung walls. Air containing carbon dioxide is then breathed out.

Why do we yawn?

When you are tired and feeling sleepy, you probably yawn. This is because your body is trying to take a deep breath to get more oxygen into your lungs.

What are hiccups?

Hiccups are caused when the muscle called the diaphragm contracts very suddenly. No-one really knows why this sometimes happens.

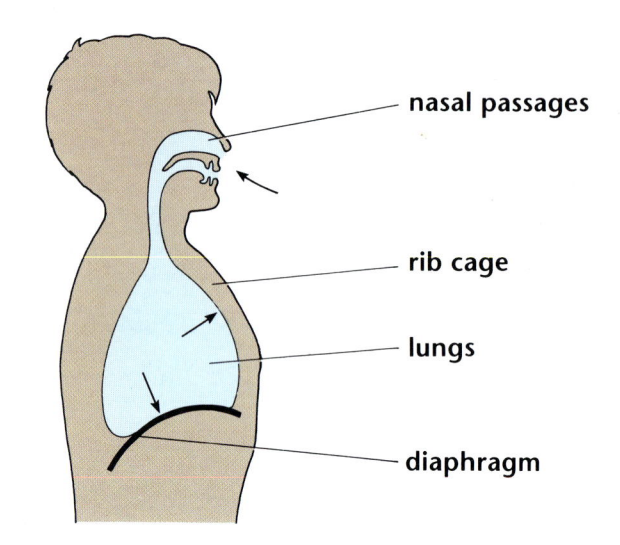

Breathing in As you breathe in your rib cage rises. A muscle called the diaphragm tightens and contracts. Your lungs expand and air rushes in through your mouth and nose to fill your lungs.

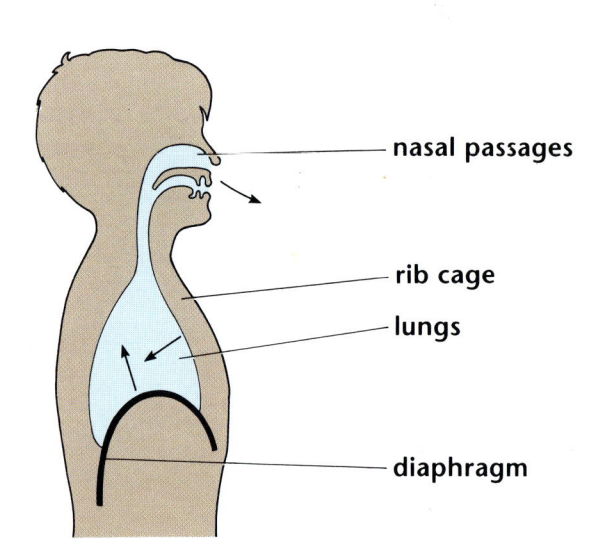

Breathing out As you breathe out your rib cage falls. The diaphragm muscle relaxes and loosens. Your lungs get smaller and some of the air in your lungs is pushed out through your nose and mouth.

Breathing problems

Like all other organs of the body, the lungs can become diseased. Many breathing problems are caused by smoking. People who smoke are more likely to develop breathing problems than non-smokers.

Smokers are more likely to develop the disease **lung cancer** than non-smokers. Lung cancer is usually fatal. You can smoke without even knowing it. Being in the same room as someone who is smoking means you are breathing smoke into your lungs. This is called passive smoking and it can be very dangerous. You can get lung cancer from passive smoking.

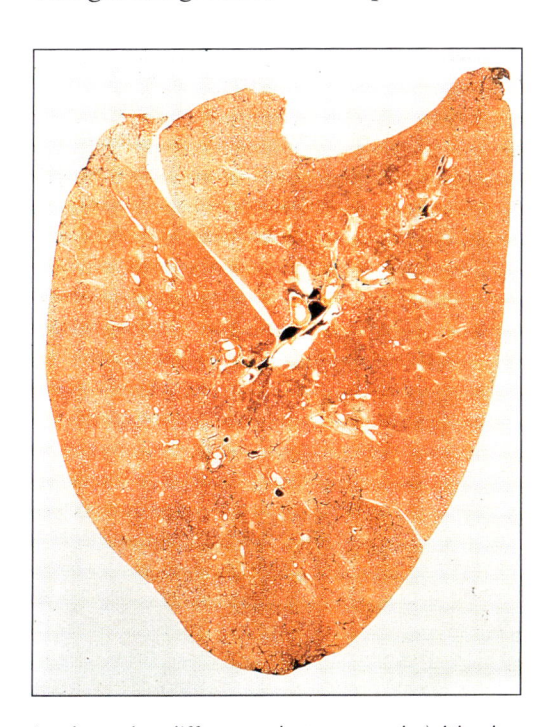

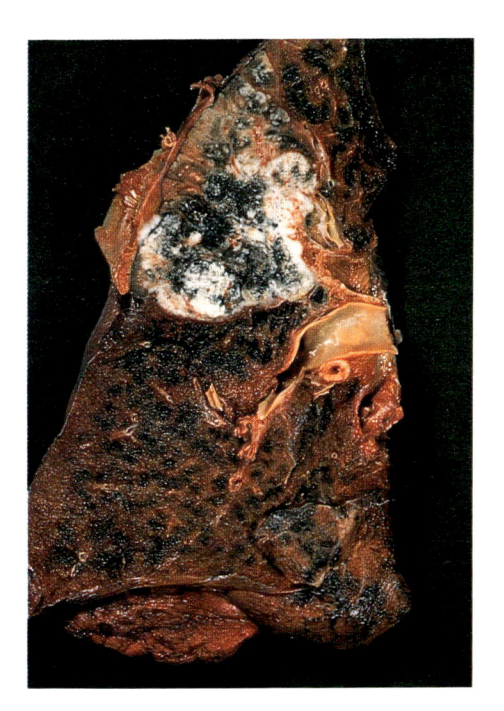

Look at the difference between a healthy lung and a smoker's lung.

🍎 **An adult's healthy lungs can hold about five litres of air, if the adult is healthy and does not smoke.**

🍎 **Focus**   breathe   oxygen   carbon dioxide   lung   blood   lung cancer

YOUR BODY

Eating to live

Why do we eat?

Everything you do needs a supply of **energy**. Walking, running, and even sleeping all need a supply of energy. Energy comes from the **food** we eat. **Nutrients** in food repair damaged body cells and help new cells to grow. The body uses nutrients for growth and for mending damaged cells. They also provide the body with energy.

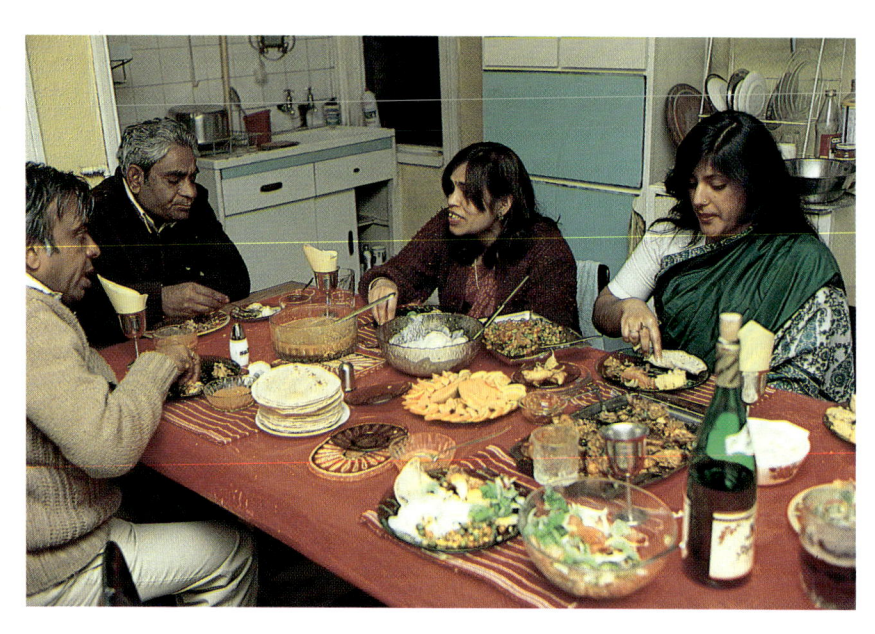

Food is the fuel that supplies you with energy.

Food mixing

Before the food you eat can do anything useful it must dissolved. When it is a liquid it can pass into your **bloodstream**. Your bloodstream then carries it to your body cells. This food mixing process is called **digestion**. Digestion takes place in the digestive system.

Food in your stomach

Food you have eaten stays in your stomach for several hours. Your stomach can easily hold a whole meal.

🍎 **Most of the digestion process does *not* take place in the stomach.**

Why does your stomach rumble?

Sometimes when you are hungry or you smell food, your stomach rumbles. This is because your stomach is preparing for the arrival of food by making extra juices for digestion.

Mouth:
your teeth chew and break up food. Liquid called saliva makes the food wet and slippery in your mouth. Saliva starts the digestion process.

Oesophagus:
a tube which squeezes food from the mouth to the stomach.

Stomach:
the digestion process continues

Small intestine:
most digestion takes place in the small intestine. Digested food (containing nutrients) passes into the bloodstream to be carried around your body

large intestine

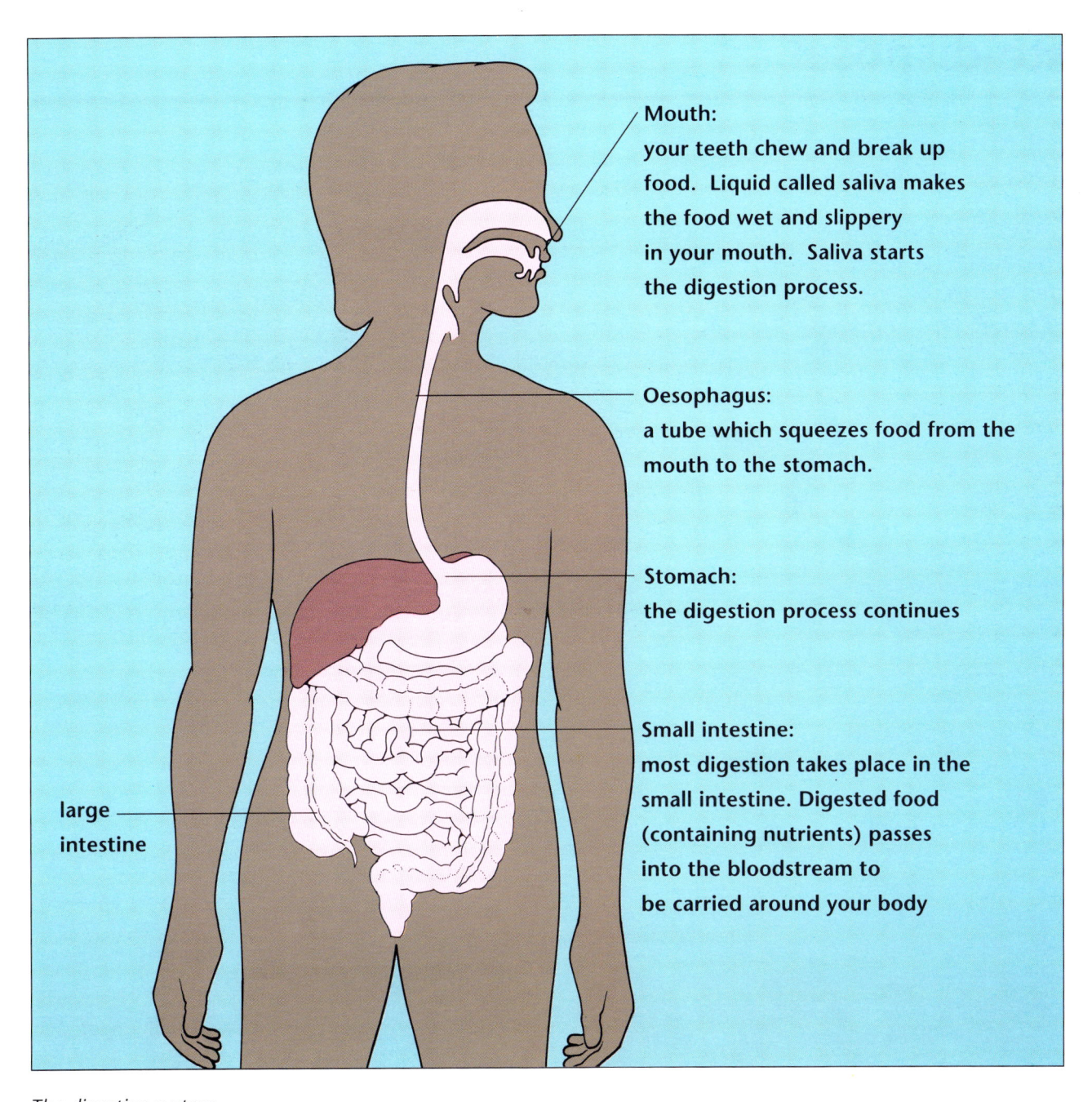

The digestive system

🍎 Your small intestine is more than 5 m long, but just 2-3 cm wide.

🍎 **Focus**   energy   food   nutrient   bloodstream   digestion

YOUR BODY

Waste disposal

Your body cannot digest all of the food you eat. You already know that some of the food is digested and passes into your body cells. **Food** that is not digested has to be removed. This is the solid **waste** your body has to get rid of.

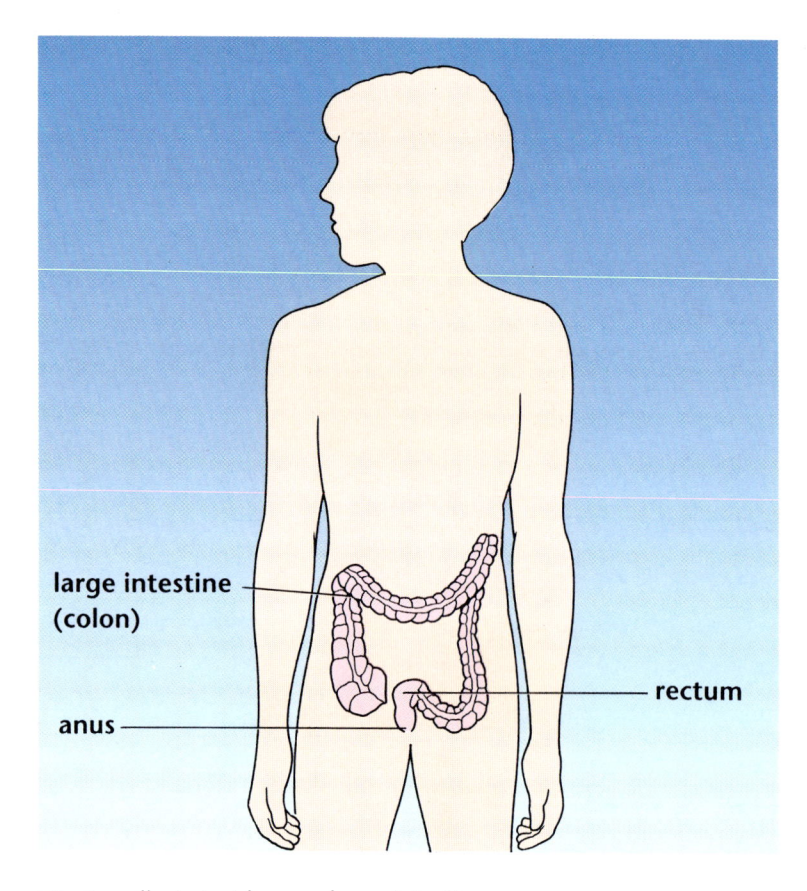

Waste collects inside your large intestine.

Inside the large intestine

Water is removed from waste in the large intestine. Waste is a soft solid called faeces. These remain at the end of the large intestine in a place called the rectum. Waste leaves your body through the anus when you go to the toilet.

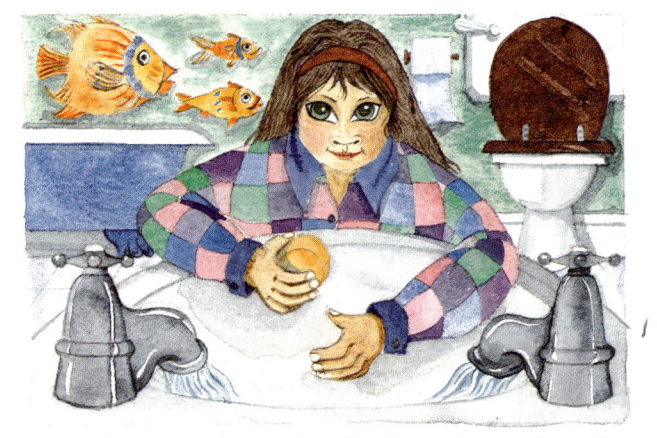

Remember to wash your hands after going to the toilet.

Liquid waste

You know that your **cells** also make waste inside your body. This waste is separate from waste made during digestion. The waste from cells is carried by blood in your **bloodstream** to your kidneys.

Your kidneys have the job of **filtering** and cleaning the blood to remove the waste. After cleaning, a watery waste fluid is left. This is called urine. Urine collects inside your bladder.

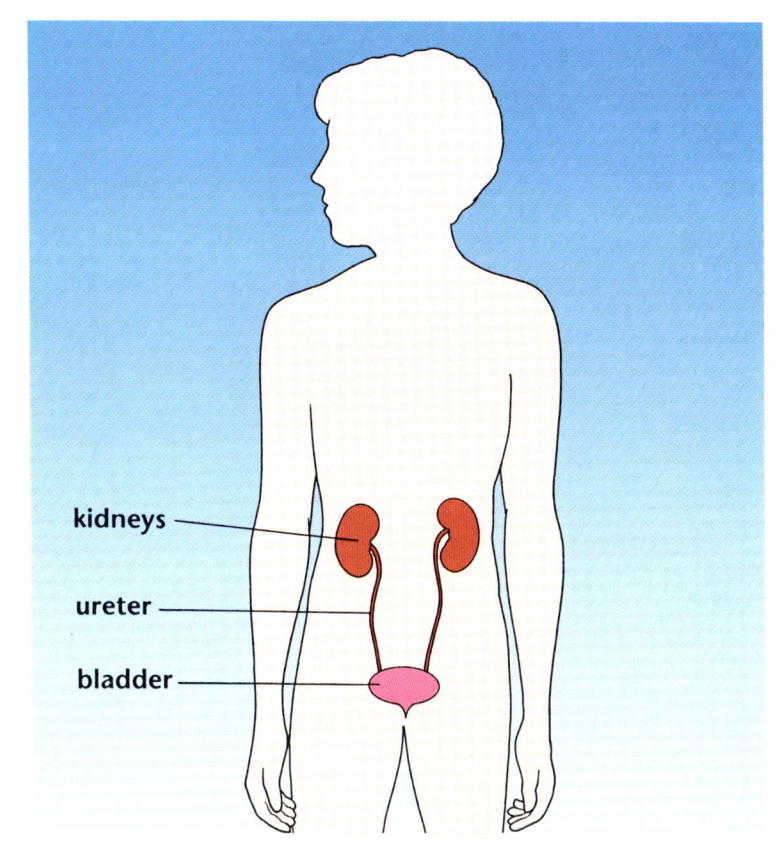

Waste liquid called urine trickles down tubes called ureters to your bladder.

What is your bladder?

Your bladder is like a stretchy bag. As it fills with urine, it gets bigger. Urine leaves your body each time you pass water into the toilet.

🍎 **In Britain, an average person gets rid of about 125 g of faeces each day.**

🍎 **Focus**   food   waste   cell   bloodstream   filtering

YOUR BODY

Blood of life

Your bloodstream is the transport system for your whole body. It carries supplies which are essential for life. Water, food, and oxygen are all carried in the bloodstream. It also removes some waste material.

What is blood?

Blood is made up of **red blood cells** and **white blood cells**. These cells all float in a yellowish liquid called **plasma**. Plasma carries carbon dioxide back to your lungs so it can be breathed out.

Red blood cells

Red blood cells contain a substance called **haemoglobin**. It is haemoglobin which gives blood its red colour. Haemoglobin has the job of carrying the oxygen supply. Oxygen enters the body through the lungs and is picked up by the haemoglobin. It is then carried to every living cell in your body.

White blood cells

You have fewer white blood cells than red blood cells. For every 1,000 red cells you have about two white blood cells. The main job of the white blood cells is to fight the germs which can make you ill. White blood cells can change shape and surround a germ to fight it. Your body can make more white blood cells if they are needed to fight germs when you become ill.

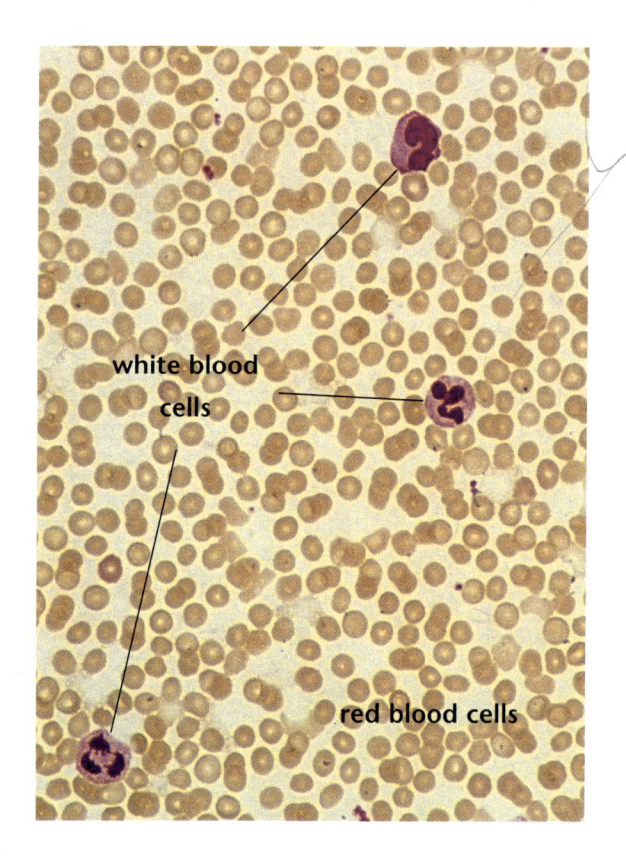

*Red blood cells are smaller than white blood cells, but there are far more of them. White blood cells are part of the body's **defence system**.*

Blood types

In humans, there are four main blood types. These are called *groups A, B, AB,* and *O.* If a person is injured in an accident they could lose a lot of blood. Doctors must be careful to find the patient's correct **blood group**.

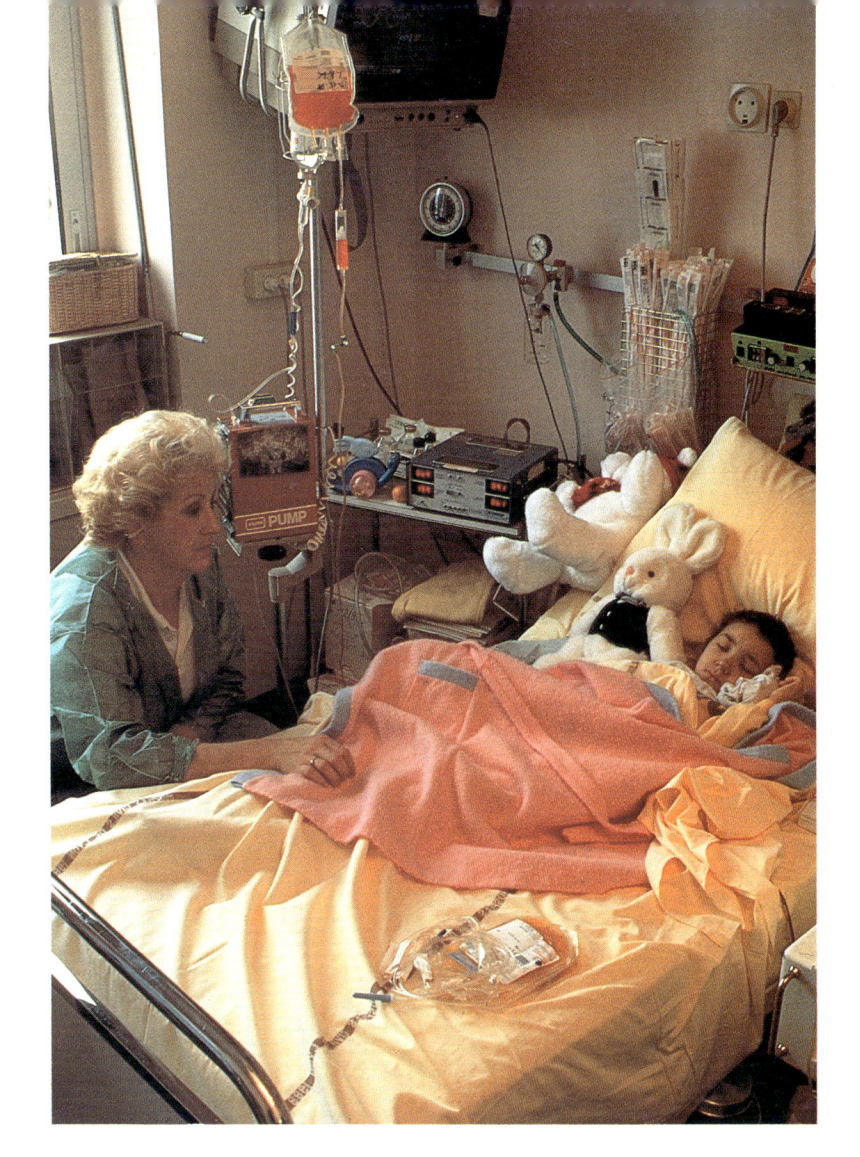

The correct match of blood group is essential if doctors need to replace blood following an accident or operation.

Haemophilia

Sometimes boys are born with a blood disease called haemophilia. For people with haemophilia, even a small cut in the skin can be dangerous. It is dangerous because it is very difficult to stop the bleeding. Doctors are able to help sufferers, who must be careful to avoid cutting themselves.

🍎 **A red blood cell lives for about four months. In that time it travels around your body about 17,000 times!**

🍎 **Focus**

bloodstream

red blood cell

white blood cell

plasma

haemoglobin

defence system

blood group

YOUR BODY

The body's pump

Your **heart** is like a machine pumping blood around your whole body. The heart is at the centre of your blood system. It controls how the oxygen-rich blood travels to your body cells. It also controls how used blood is returned to your lungs to get rid of carbon dioxide as waste and to pick up more oxygen.

Your heart is divided into four 'rooms', two on each side. Each side of your heart has the job of delivering and receiving blood. The receiving rooms are called the left and right **atriums**. *The delivering rooms are called the left and right* **ventricles**.

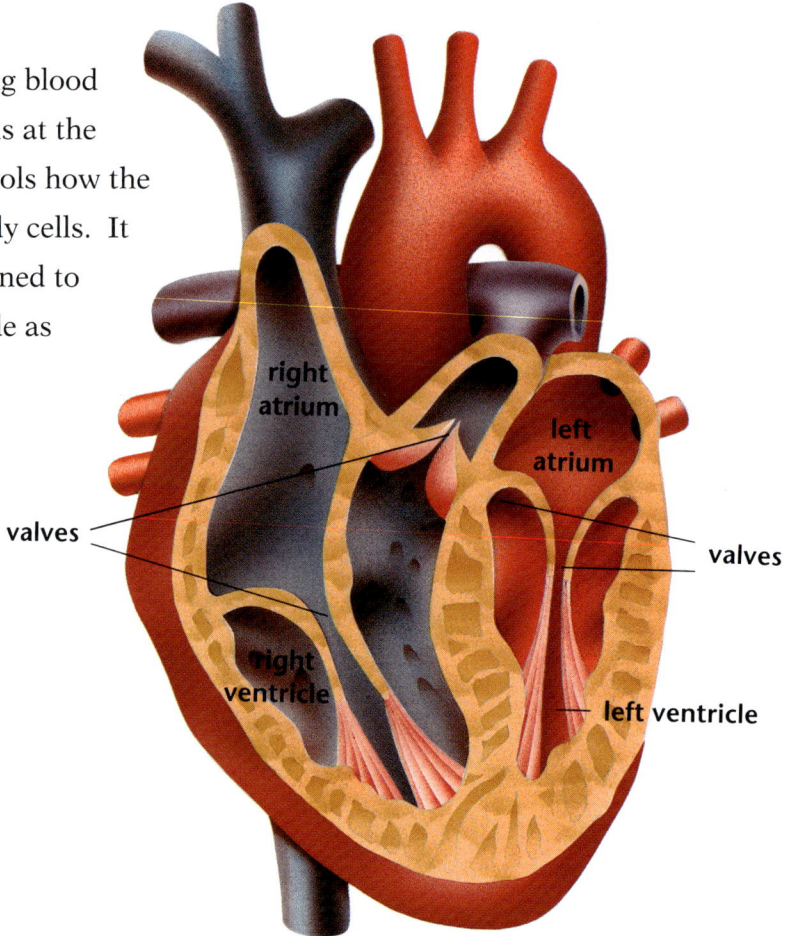

'Used' blood

One 'room' is called the right atrium. This is where blood returning to the lungs collects. This is blood that has already been around the body. it has used up its oxygen and is going to the lungs for more. The used blood goes from the right atrium to the right ventricle. It is them pumped to the lungs for a fresh supply of oxygen.

'Fresh' blood

Fresh oxygen-rich blood collects in the left atrium. It passes to the left ventricle and is pumped around the body to deliver oxygen.

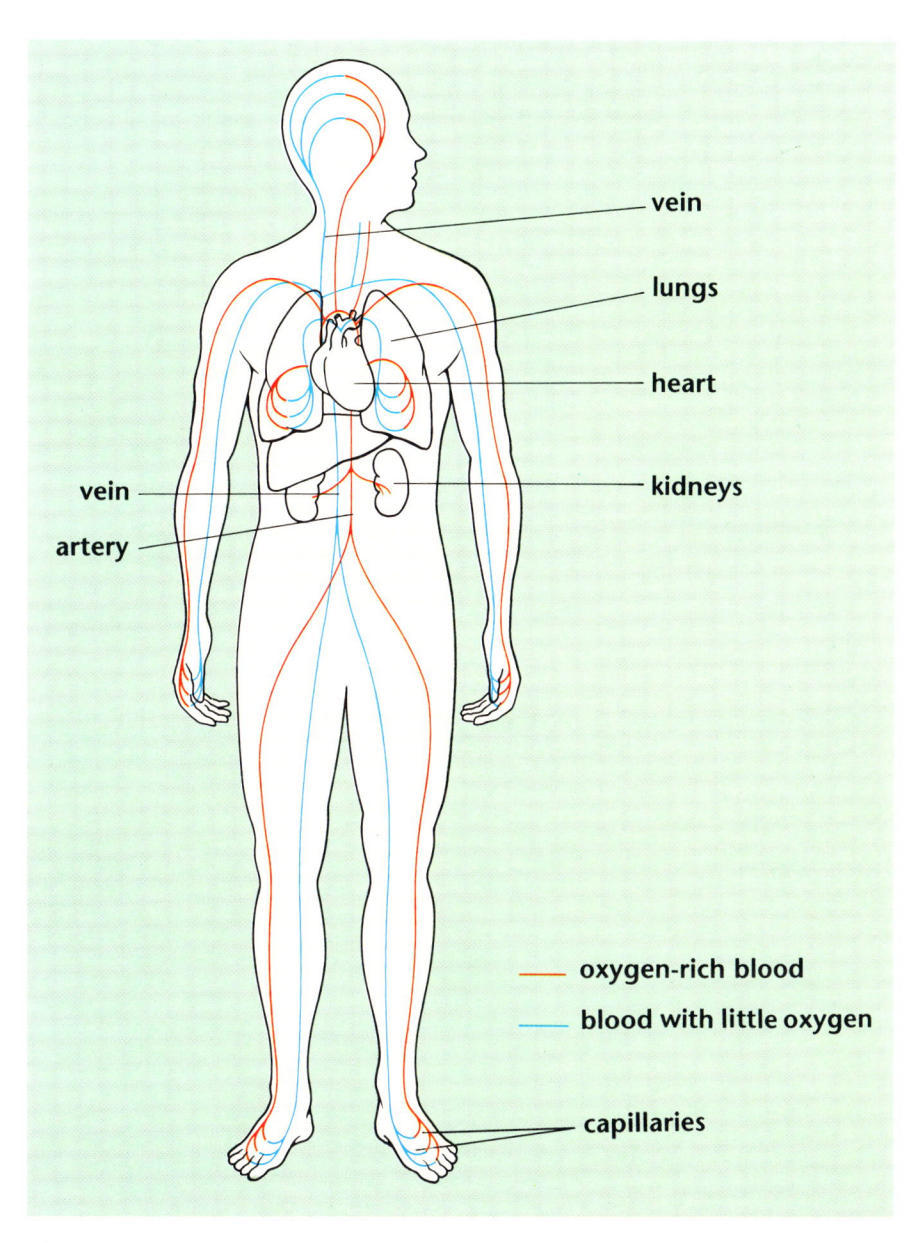

Blood is pumped around your body in a network of tubes called **arteries**, **veins**, and **capillaries**. Oxygen-rich blood is pumped around your body in arteries and capillaries. Blood with little oxygen but a lot of carbon dioxide is returned to the lungs in veins.

🍎 **Your heart is about the size of a clenched fist.**

🍎 **Focus**   heart   atrium   ventricle   artery   capillary   vein

YOUR BODY

Keeping control

Imagine how difficult everything would be if you had no control over your body. You wouldn't be able to walk, talk, play, eat, or do anything when you wanted to.

What is the brain?

Your **brain** is very sensitive and quite easily damaged. It is protected inside your skull which is like a very strong box. Between your skull and your brain there is a layer of liquid. This absorbs any shocks if you bang or shake your head.

The body's telephone lines

Your brain is linked to other parts of your body by **nerves**. These are a bit like telephone lines which send messages to and from the brain.

These messages are sorted out in the brain and instructions are sent back to parts of the body along the nerves. This is the body's **nervous system**.

Spinal cord

Your **spinal cord** is a bundle of nerves which goes down your back inside the spine. The smaller nerves go from the spinal cord to other parts of your body.

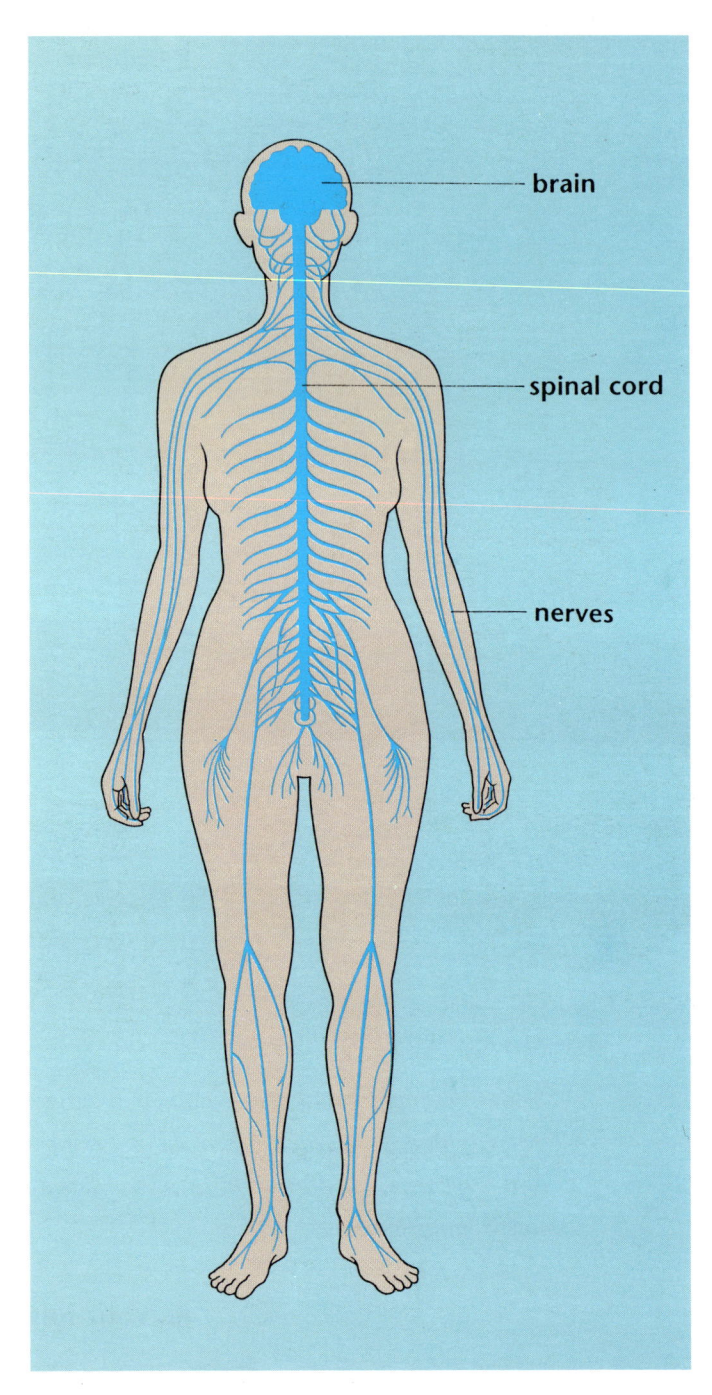

Your nervous system is made up of your brain, your spinal cord, and many nerves.

speech

touch

hearing

thoughts and feelings

movement

Your brain has several different areas. Each one is responsible for different actions or skills.

sight

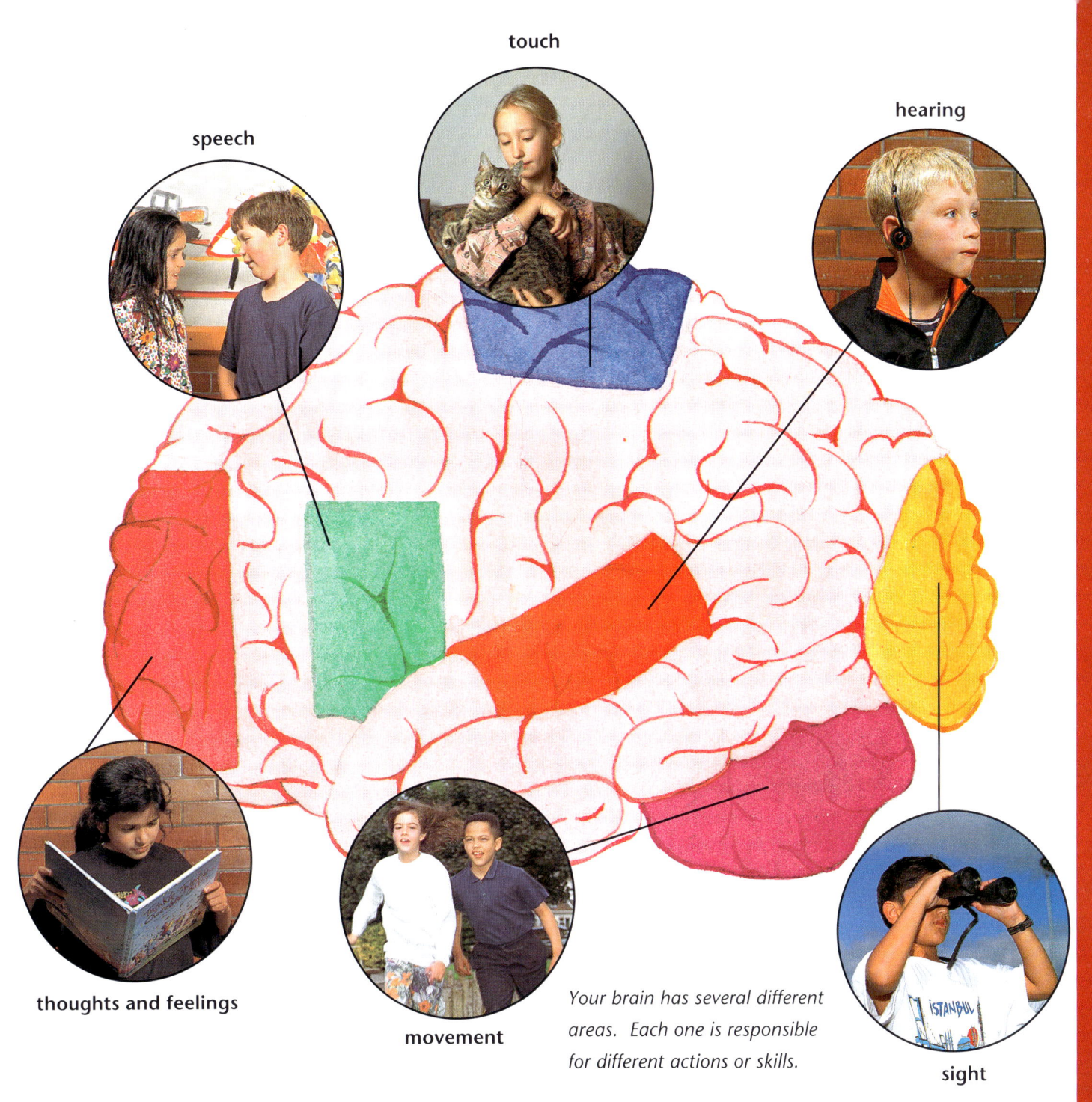

Reflex action

If you sit with crossed legs, and a friend taps you just below the knee, your foot will move up sharply. You cannot stop it. This is a reflex action. You have no control over a reflex action.

🍎 **Focus**   brain   nerve   nervous system   spinal cord

19

YOUR BODY

Your framework of bones

The **skeleton** is a framework of bones that **supports** your body. Without it you would collapse!

It is easy to think of your bones as things that are completely solid like metal bars. In fact, your bones are living material. They need a blood supply just like the rest of your body. All through your life, your height will depend upon the size of your skeleton.

When you were born you had about 350 bones. When you become fully grown up you will have 206. This is because lots of tiny bones join up as you grow.

Bones for protection

Some of your bones **protect** other, softer parts of your body. Your rib cage is made up of pairs of ribs. Ribs protect your heart and lungs. Your spine is a collection of bones running down your back. Your spine protects your spinal cord. Your skull protects your brain. The skull is made up of 29 bones. Most bones in the skull are joined firmly together. The jaw bone is the only one that can move.

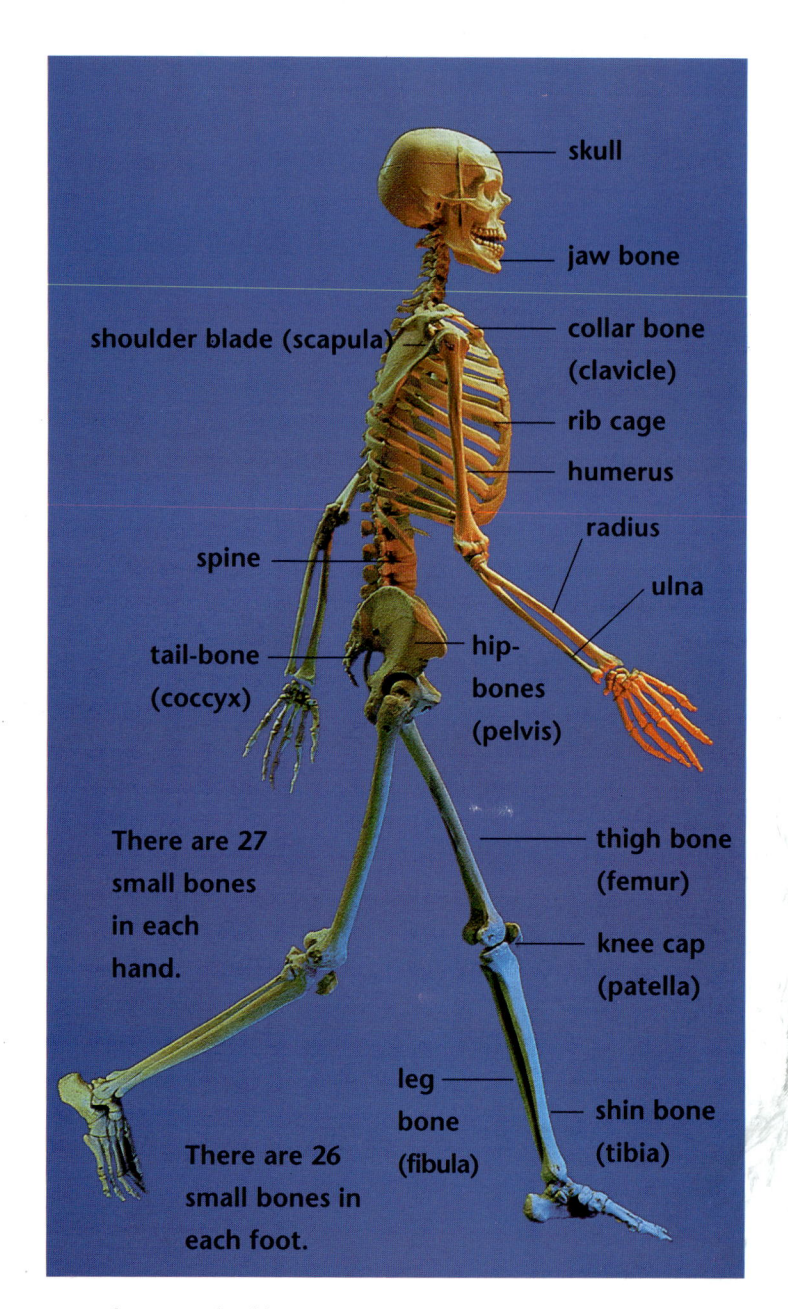

Labels on skeleton diagram: skull, jaw bone, shoulder blade (scapula), collar bone (clavicle), rib cage, humerus, radius, spine, ulna, tail-bone (coccyx), hip-bones (pelvis), thigh bone (femur), knee cap (patella), leg bone (fibula), shin bone (tibia)

There are 27 small bones in each hand.

There are 26 small bones in each foot.

Your framework of bones

20

Bones meet at the joints

Some of the bones in your body meet at **joints**. You have different kinds of joints for the different movements your body needs to make. Your elbow joint is called a hinge joint. It can move up and down in one direction only, like the hinge of a door. The joint at your hip is a ball and socket joint. It can move in *all* directions.

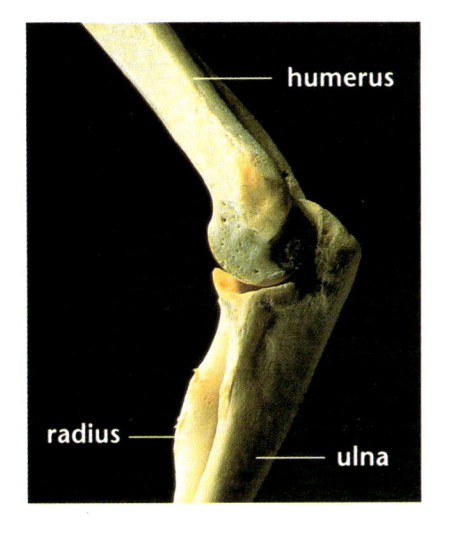

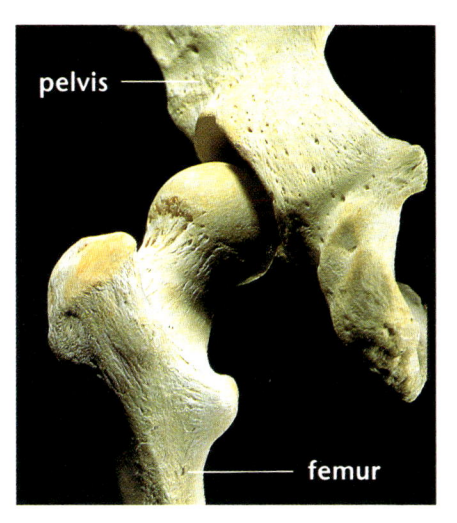

Joints help your body to move

How broken bones mend

A broken bone begins to heal itself very quickly. New bone starts to grow from the broken ends. After about six weeks, the bone will be completely healed. A broken bone in your arm or leg can heal much faster than an adult's.

If you break your arm or leg, the doctor will put it into a plaster cast. This is so it cannot move, and the bone can heal.

🍎 **The tallest groups of people in the world are found in Central Africa. The average height of some tribes is more than 1.83 m tall.**

🍎 **Focus**

skeleton
support
protect
joint

YOUR BODY

Every move you make

Every move you make uses many **muscles**. You use them to bend, to run, to walk, to breathe, and even to open and close your eyes.

Like the rest of your body, muscles are made up of **cells**. You have special muscle cells that make some muscles into a mass of string-like fibres. Muscles can only pull, they cannot push.

Your muscles develop in strength according to what you do. If you try and lift a heavy weight when you are not used to it, you could strain your muscles. Weight-lifters develop huge muscles in order to succeed in their sport.

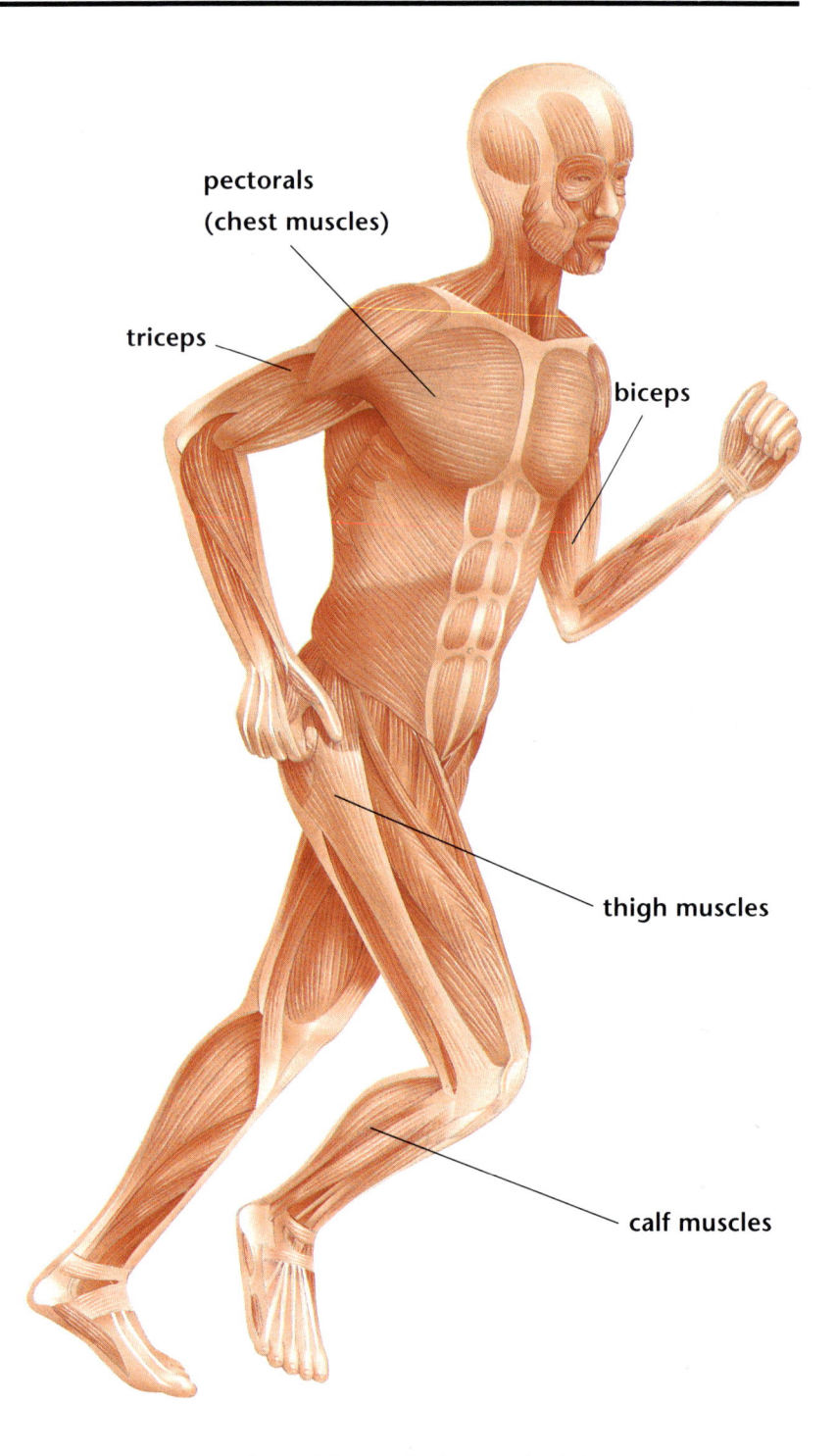

There are more than 650 muscles in your body.

Skeletal muscles

You have more than 600 **skeletal muscles**. These are muscles fixed on to the skeleton just below the skin. You are able to control the movements of skeletal muscles, so they are sometimes called **voluntary muscles**. Each time you run, walk, throw a ball, or make any voluntary movement, you are using your skeletal muscles.

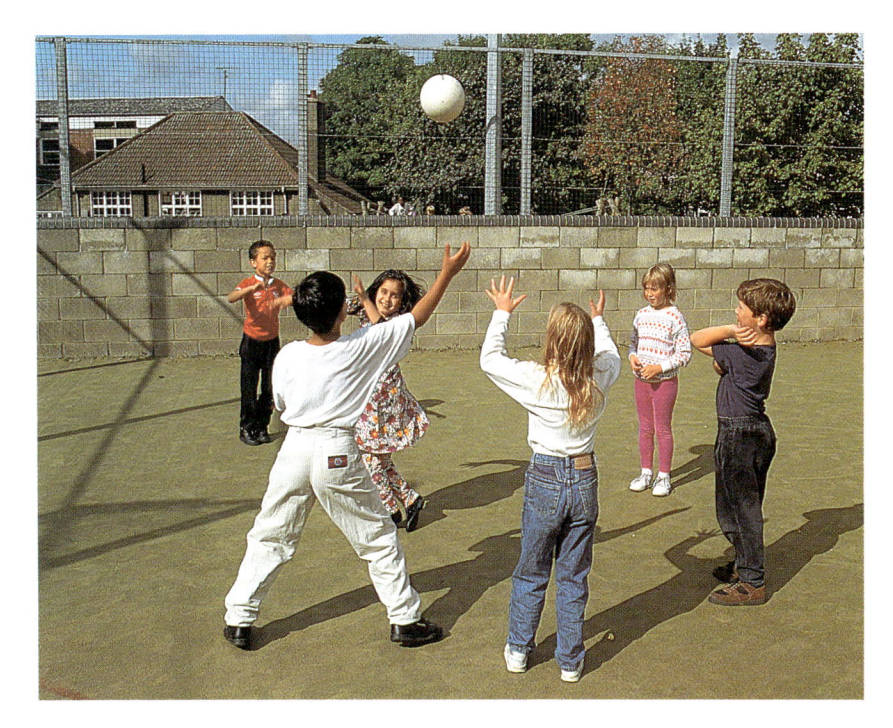

All of your movements use your skeletal muscles.

Smooth muscles

Smooth muscles are muscles that work automatically all of the time. They control the inside of your body. They can also be called **involuntary muscles**. Smooth muscles have jobs which include forcing food through the digestive system.

Cardiac muscle

The third type of muscle is **cardiac muscle**. This is the muscle of your heart. Its job is to pump the blood around your body all of the time.

🍎 You use more than 200 different muscles each time you take a step. You only have one muscle behind each ear to help wiggle your ears! Only a few people are able to use their 'ear wiggling muscles'. Can you?

🍎 **Focus**

muscle

cell

skeletal muscle

voluntary muscle

smooth muscle

involuntary muscle

cardiac muscle

YOUR SENSES

Look and listen

On your way to school, you might have to cross a road. You stop at the kerb. You look both ways, and you listen. Looking and listening use your **senses** of **sight** and **hearing**. Senses pick up **messages**. These messages can warn you about dangers, and can help to keep you safe.

Your sense of sight

Your eyes control your sense of sight. The part of the eye which can be seen is small. Your eye is really the size of a table-tennis ball.

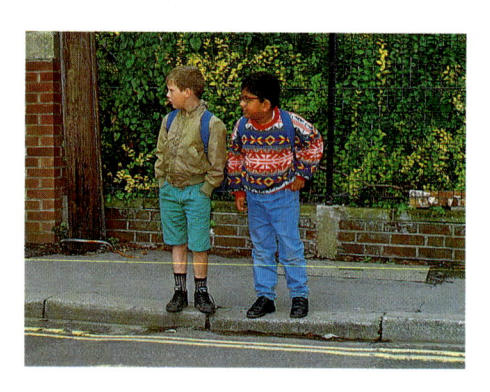

Eyes work a bit like cameras. When you look at an object or a view, light passes through the pupil. The lens in your eye focuses the picture, making it clear. The picture of the object or view appears upside down on the retina at the back of the eye.

The retina has special cells which are sensitive to light. These special cells send messages along the optic nerve to your brain. Your brain makes sense of the messages and turns the picture the right way up.

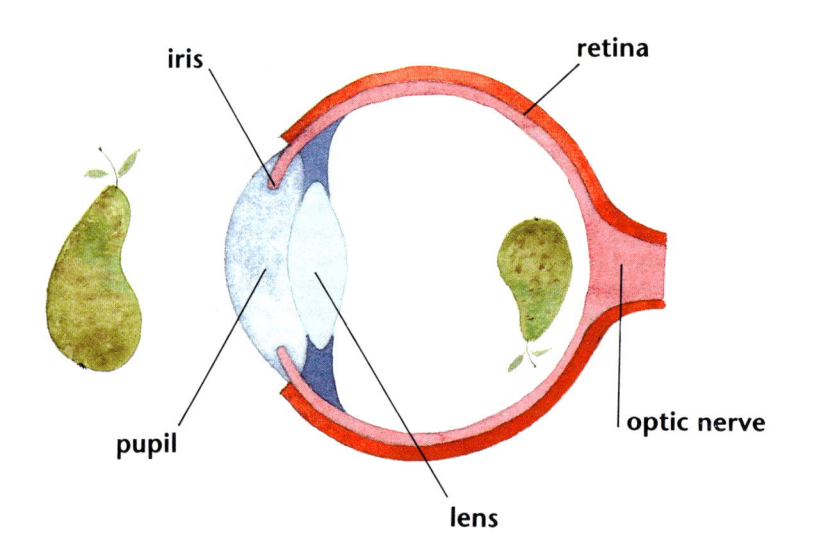

The senses of sight and hearing help you to cross the road safely.

Your eyes produce pictures that are upside down. Your brain turns them the right way up.

24

Your sense of hearing

Sounds are picked up by your outer ear. The outer ear is the part you can see. Sounds pass to the middle ear, where they make the skin of the eardrum move backwards and forwards or **vibrate**. The vibrations are passed through three tiny bones, and then into a liquid-filled tube in the inner ear called the cochlea. It is shaped like a spiral. The nerves in the cochlea change the vibrations into messages to send along to the brain.

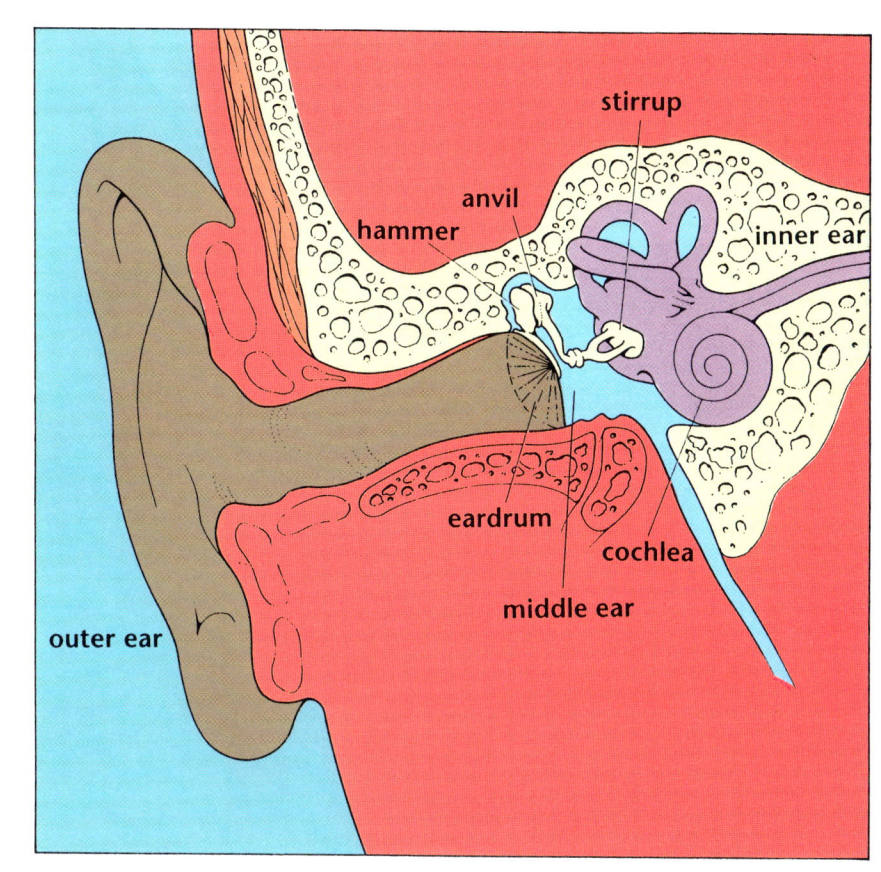

Your ear is made up of three main sections called the outer, middle, and inner ear.

🍎 If you spin around and make yourself dizzy you can lose your balance. This is because the liquid in your cochlea is swirling around quickly. The messages to your brain become confused. Your ears are important in helping your body to balance.

🍎 **Focus**   sense   hearing   sight   message   vibrate

YOUR SENSES

Smells good, tastes good

If you have ever smelt a cake baking in the oven, you'll know how good smells can be. When the cake is baked and you taste it, you'll know how great tastes can be! **Smell** and **taste** are two more of your **senses**.

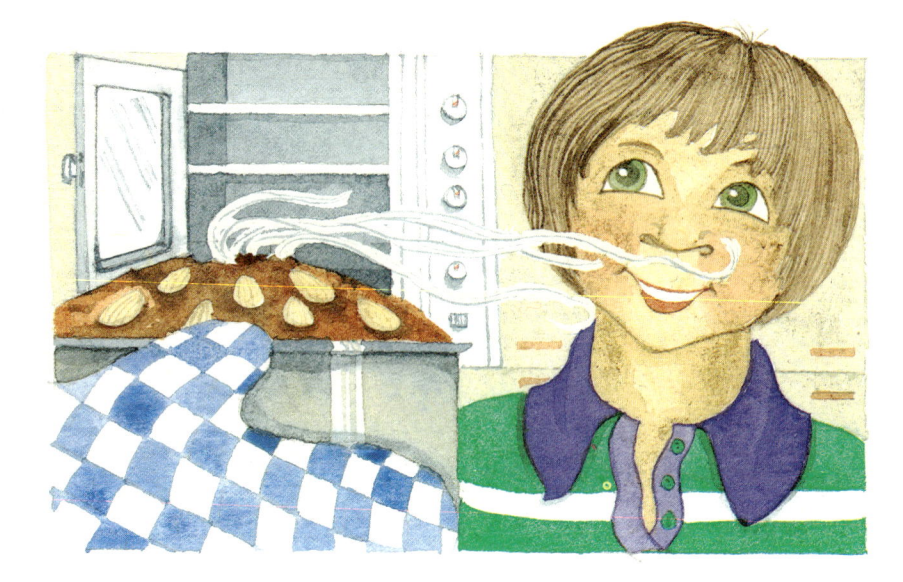

Smells can sometimes be really good.

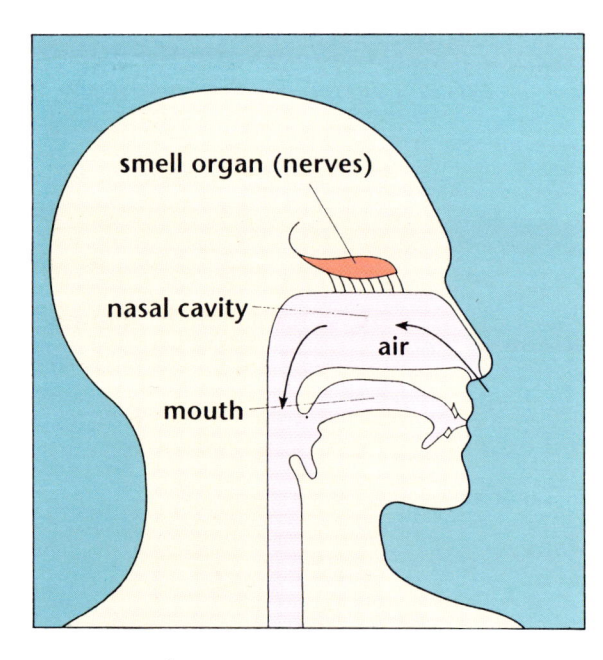

The parts of your nose

Your sense of smell

Your nose can detect thousands of different smells. Your nose is also used to breathe air in and out of your lungs. When you breathe in air through your nose it passes over a sensitive area known as the smell organ.

This area contains fine hairs and also **nerves**. The nerves pick up smells and send **messages** about those smells to your brain. Your brain uses the messages to identify the smells.

● **The most important function of your nose is to warm the air you breathe in before it reaches your lungs.**

26

How do you taste things?

When you eat something you can instantly tell if it is sweet, salty, bitter, or sour. Your tongue is very sensitive to the four tastes: salt, sour, bitter, and sweet.

Your tongue

Your tongue helps you speak by shaping words. It also helps you eat and taste food. There are about 3,000 taste buds on your tongue. They are sensitive cells which send messages to your brain about the tastes you experience.

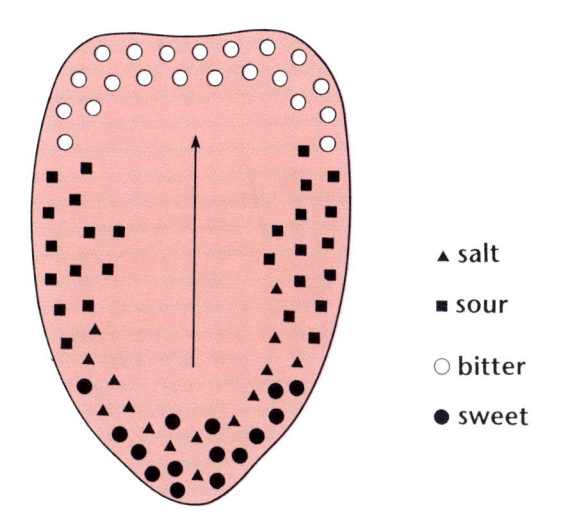

▲ salt
■ sour
○ bitter
● sweet

This taste map of your tongue shows where the four tastes are detected.

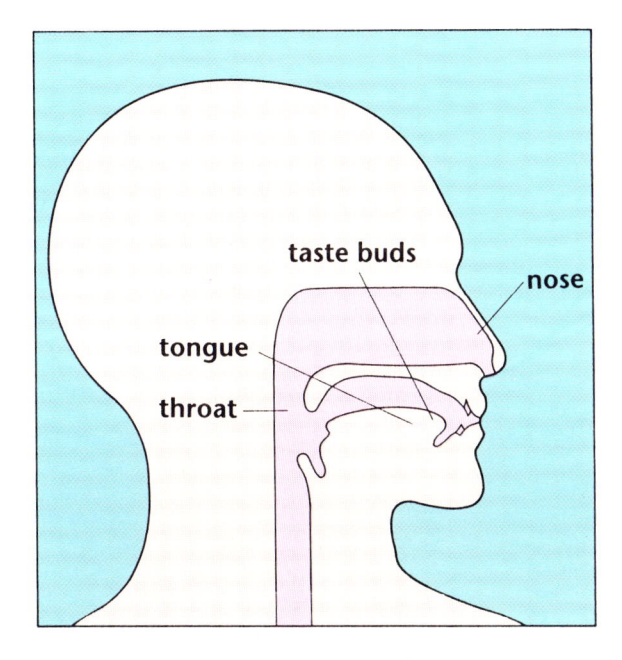

Messages pass from the taste buds on your tongue to your brain.

You smell what you eat

If you have a cold with a blocked up nose, food doesn't taste too good. This is because when you eat, much of what you think you taste is really smell. Your sense of smell is far more powerful than your sense of taste.

● **Focus**   smell   taste   sense   nerve   message

YOUR SENSES

Skin deep

When you **touch** something with your hands, you feel different textures. If you fall over in the playground, you'll feel the rough texture of the gravel. When you stroke a cat or dog, you can feel the smooth, silky texture of its fur. Touch is one of your **senses**.

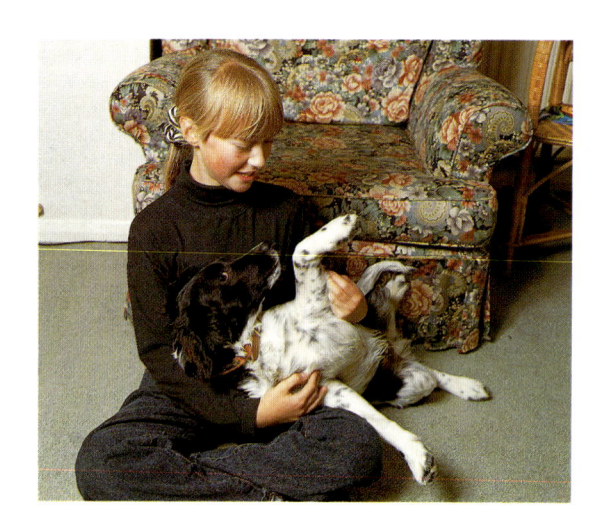

Your skin uses the sense of touch to feel different things.

Skin

Your skin is the largest part of your body. It must be, because it covers up everything else. Skin is made up of millions of skin cells. Most of your sense of touch is in your skin. It is full of **nerve endings** which collect **messages** about surfaces and temperature, for example. These messages are sent to your brain to be understood.

Your skin does an amazing number of things:

- it keeps your insides in!
- it is waterproof
- it bends and stretches
- it keeps germs out
- it sweats when you are hot
- it tells you about temperature, shape, and texture of things that you touch
- it repairs itself

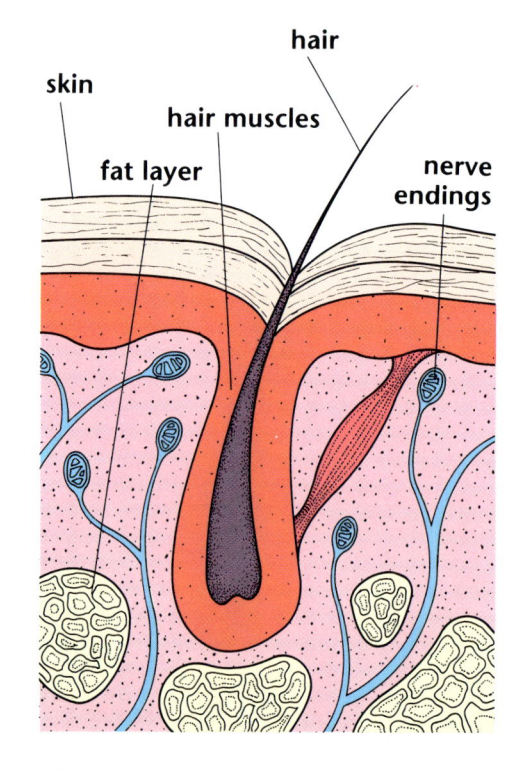

The make-up of your skin

What happens when you sweat?

The hotter you get, the more you **sweat**. Sweating helps you cool down because the sweat evaporates from your skin and removes heat from your body.

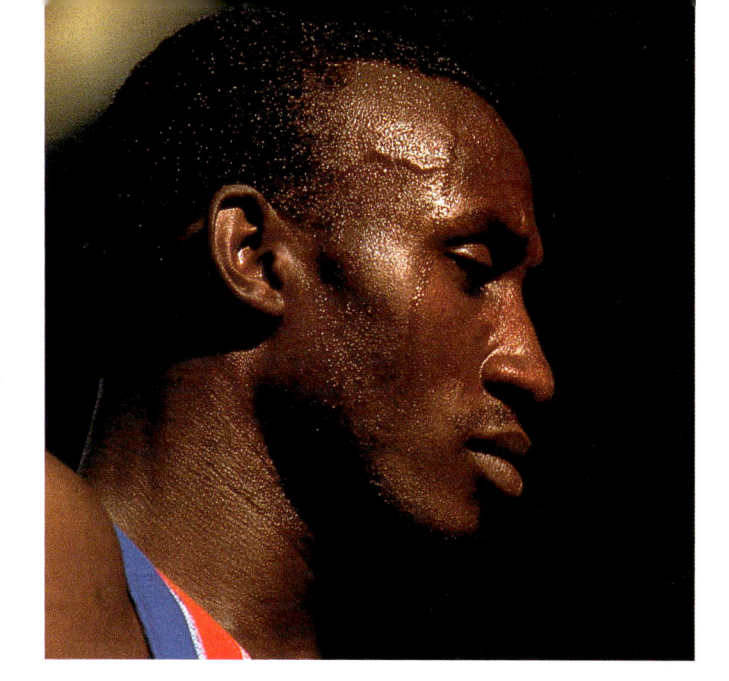

Sweat is salty water made in your skin.

Your skin repairs itself

Your body starts to repair cuts or grazes as soon as they happen. Blood cells make the bleeding stop and the blood clot. The clot becomes a protective covering over the wound. This is called a scab. Skin cells grow beneath the scab, which soon falls off. The healed cut will be covered with new skin cells.

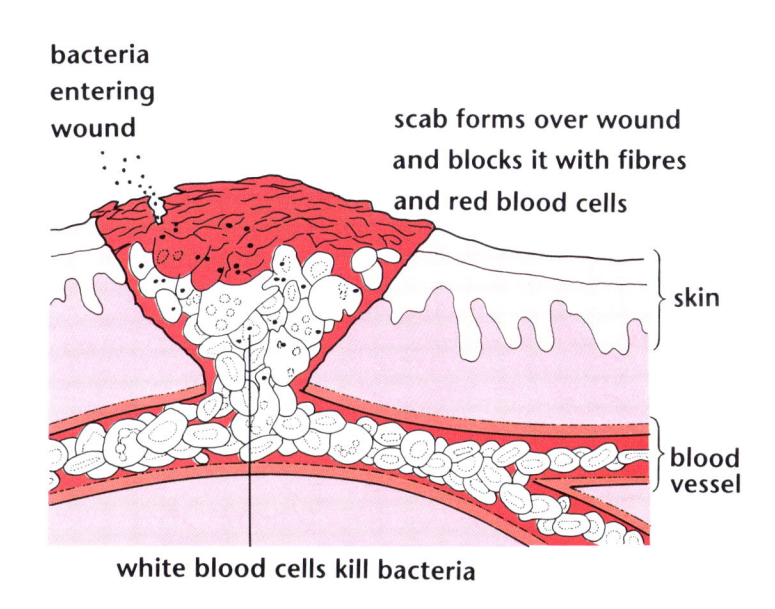

bacteria entering wound

scab forms over wound and blocks it with fibres and red blood cells

skin

blood vessel

white blood cells kill bacteria

How a scab forms

🍎 **Millions of skin cells are lost and replaced every day. Your body is constantly making more.**

🍎 **Focus**   touch   sense   nerve ending   message   sweat

● KEEPING HEALTHY

What you eat

What kinds of food do you enjoy eating?

Do you like sweets or fruit?

Do you enjoy vegetables or meat?

What are your favourite foods?

All of the foods and drinks you eat make up your diet. Your **diet** will be different from that of your parents and your friends.

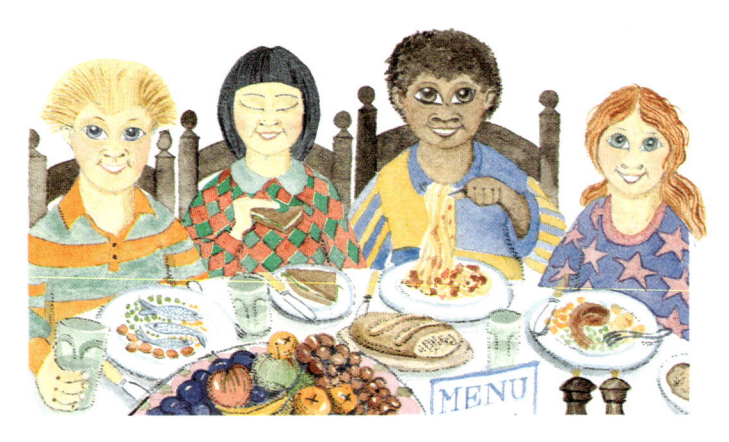

What foods do you enjoy eating?

Right or wrong foods?

Generally there are no such things as right foods and wrong foods, or good foods and bad foods. There are healthy and unhealthy diets which everyone needs to know about. Your body needs a healthy diet so that it works and grows properly.

What makes a healthy diet?

A **healthy diet** contains the **nutrients** needed by your body. Nutrients are substances in food and drink which give you **energy** and help you grow and be strong. They also help to keep you healthy, free from illness. A healthy diet should include these nutrients (together with water and fibre):

Nutrients	Some foods containing one or more of them
fat	butter, cheese, chips, milk
carbohydrate	cereals, bread, rice, potatoes, pasta
protein	meat, fish, milk, nuts
vitamins	oranges, carrots, green peppers
minerals	liver, spinach, milk
(fibre)	fruit, vegetables, cereals

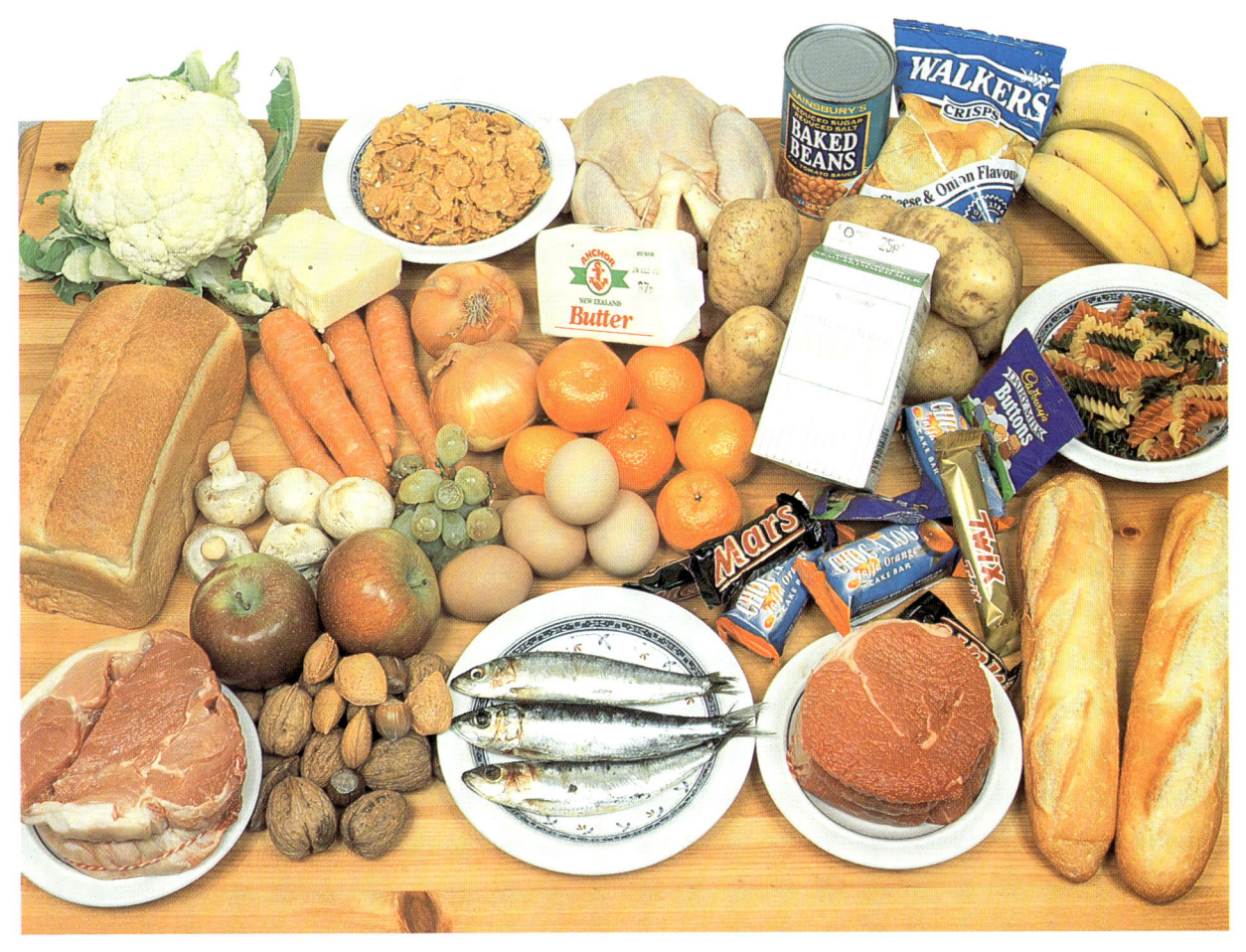

These are some of the foods which contain nutrients needed by your body.

A good balance is needed

To keep fit and healthy, a sensible balance of nutrients is needed. Try not to eat too much of any one thing, such as biscuits or crisps.

The food you eat affects your whole body. With a healthy diet the organs in your body will work properly. Your heart will stay strong and you will be able to get rid of waste regularly.

🍏 **The average person in Britain eats about half-a-tonne of food every year. This does not include drinks.**

🍏 **Focus**   diet   healthy diet   nutrient   energy

KEEPING HEALTHY

Enough to eat

Have you ever asked how long it is to dinner because you are hungry? How often have you returned home after school and complained about being starving?

You have probably felt hungry at some time, but were you really starving?

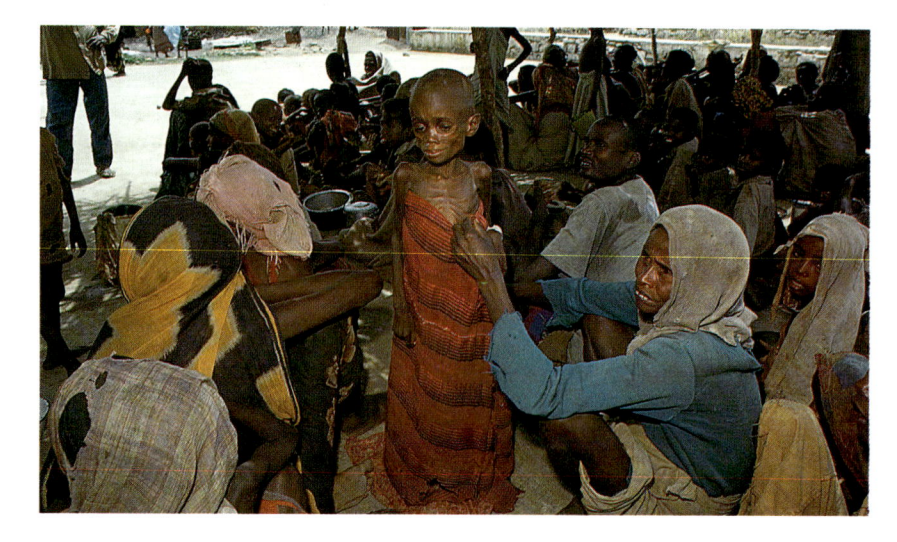

This child in Somalia is really starving.

Enough food

In some countries, people die because they don't have enough **food**. Everyone needs food to live. If you don't eat well enough, you become ill. This is called **malnutrition**. If you don't eat, you *will* die.

Famine

In poor countries it can be difficult to get enough food to eat for many reasons. These include:

- crop failure due to no rainfall, leading to drought
- crop disease
- conflicts and war
- the need to sell any food produced to pay debts

All of these things can lead to famine. **Famine** is when a whole area in a country cannot get enough food. It causes terrible suffering and many deaths.

A long life?

People who don't get enough food will not live as long as people who get the right amount. The length of time people are expected to live is called life expectancy:

- in Europe, life expectancy is about 75 years
- in Malaysia, life expectancy is about 67 years
- in Ethiopia, life expectancy is about 39 years

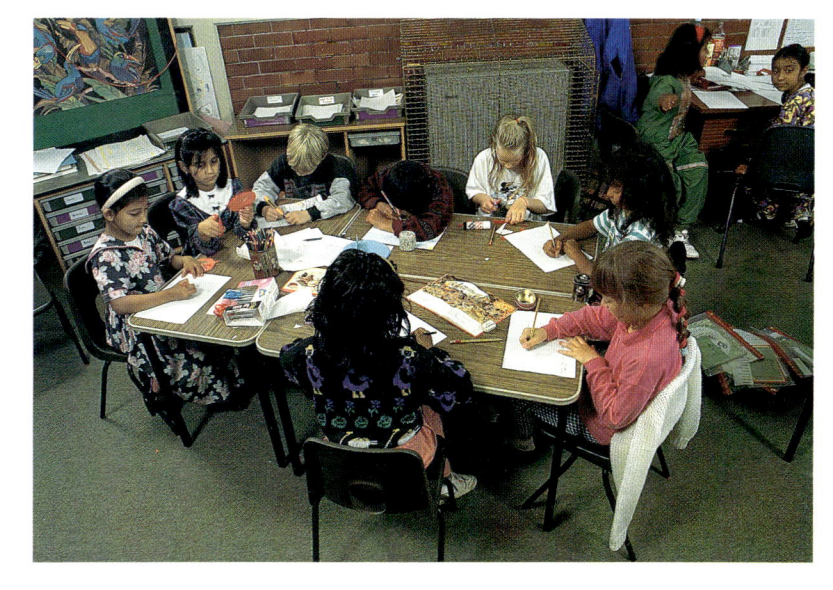

If these children have a good balanced diet, they can hope to live for about 75 years.

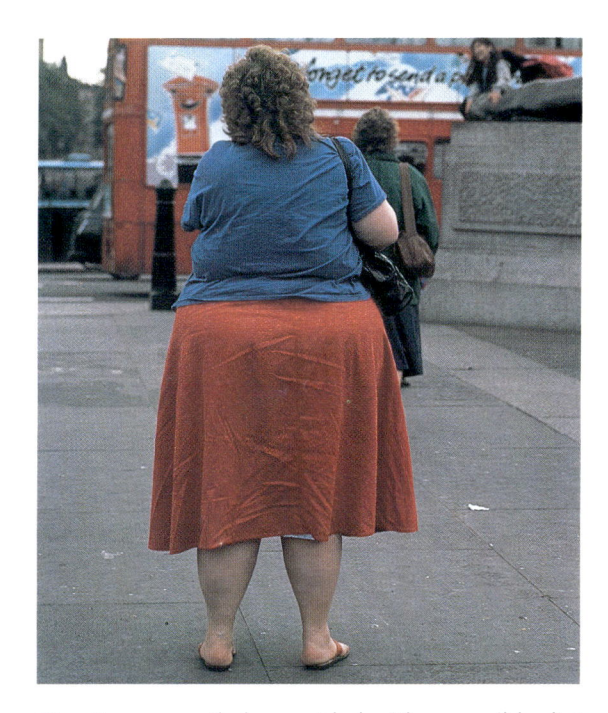

Too much food

In rich countries, eating too much food is a problem. It causes **obesity**. Someone who suffers from obesity is too fat to be healthy. Obesity can lead to early death, often through heart disease.

Too little food

In rich countries, where food may be plentiful, some people eat too little food. They may develop the slimmers' disease **anorexia nervosa**. Like obesity, this can lead to death.

Obesity can easily be avoided with a sensible diet.

Focus   food   malnutrition   famine   obesity   anorexia nervosa

KEEPING HEALTHY

Keeping clean

How often do you wash your hands?

Do you clean your teeth regularly?

Do you often take showers or have a bath?

When do you wash your hair?

If you do all of these regularly, then you know the importance of **personal hygiene**. Keeping your body clean helps to prevent illness. Many illnesses are caused by germs. **Germs** spread very quickly.

Washing your hands

Germs can easily be spread when you use your hands. You can prevent the spread of germs by washing your hands:

- after visiting the toilet
- after handling pets
- after playing outside
- before cooking and handling foods

Looking after your teeth

You should brush your teeth after every meal. Sometimes it is not possible, especially if you are away from home. If it is not you should at least brush them in the morning and again before you go to bed. You should also have regular check-ups at the dentist. Eating too much sugar and ignoring your teeth will lead to tooth decay. This is when your teeth begin to rot away, causing you painful toothache and emergency visits to the dentist!

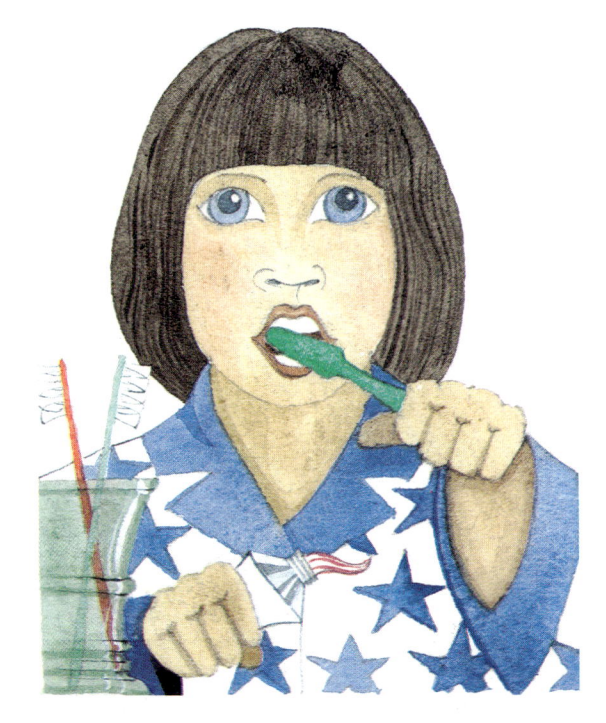

Regularly brushing your teeth is important.

Handling food

You know how important it is to wash your hands before handling food. There are several other hygienic things you can do to avoid spreading germs when handling foods:

- use clean utensils
- use clean work surfaces and chopping boards
- use clean tea towels and dish cloths
- tie back your hair if it is too long

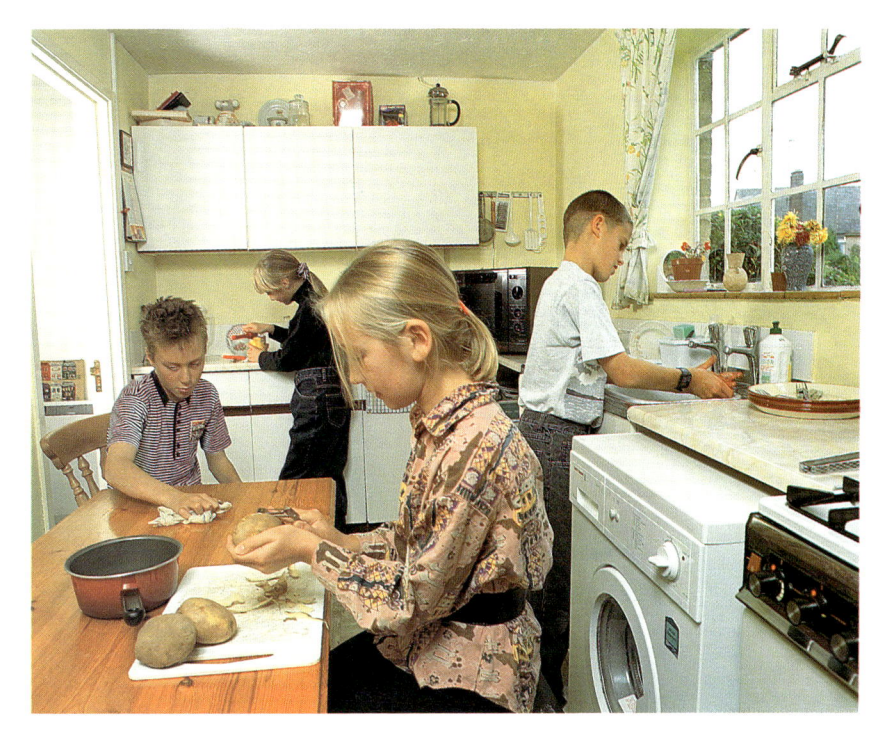

Careful handling of food prevents germs from spreading

Food poisoning

If you keep to the simple rules of hygiene and also take care when handling food, you will avoid the spread of germs on food.

Germs on food can cause food poisoning. Salmonella is a bacterium found in some foods. It can cause a serious kind of food poisoning. It will make you very sick with an upset stomach and diarrhoea.

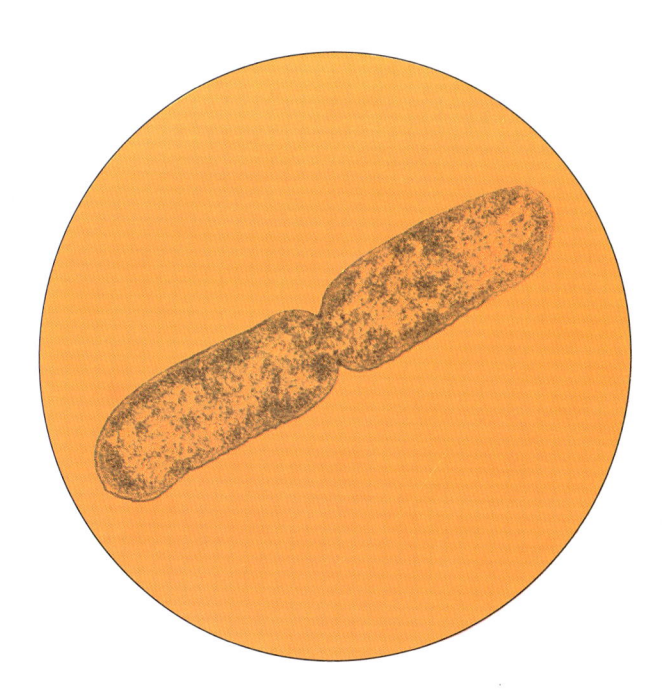

Food poisoning is caused by the spread of a bacterium called Salmonella (magnification 50,000 times).

Focus   personal hygiene   germ

KEEPING HEALTHY

Exercise and resting

Exercise is a very important part of living. Exercise helps to keep you healthy and fit. At school you exercise during games lessons, and at break times. Out of school, you might go for bike rides or walks.

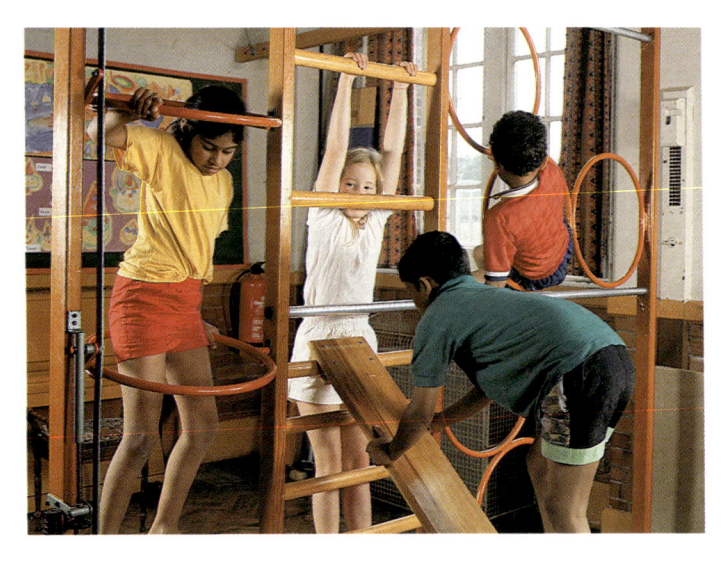

Exercise helps to keep you fit

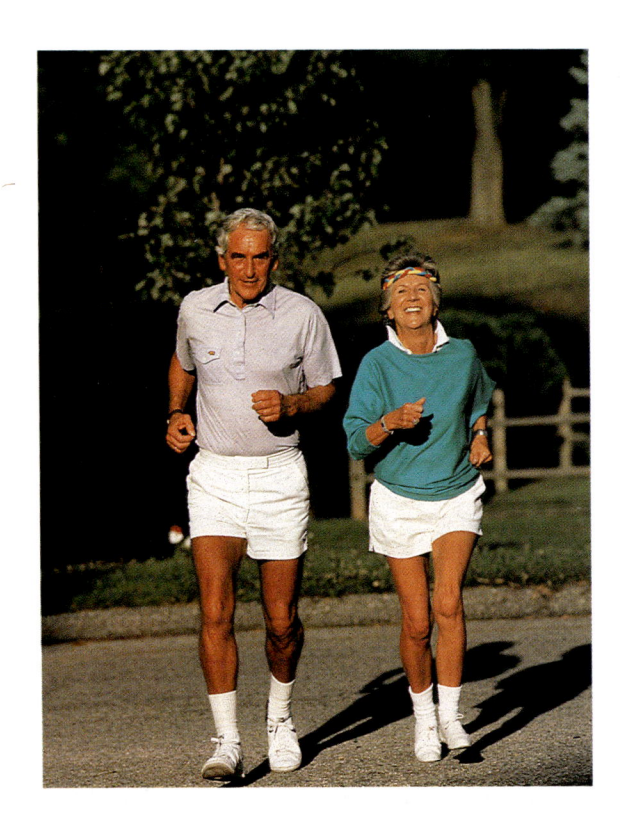

Regular exercise can lead to a healthier, longer life.

Why exercise?

If you do not take regular exercise, your muscles will get weak. Exercise helps to keep the body machine working. Your **heart** is a muscle, so it needs exercise too. When you are running or playing outdoor games, your heart will beat faster. You will get a little breathless. Your heart has to work harder pumping blood to your muscles.

Adults need to exercise

You probably run around at school and at home, enough to stay fit and healthy. Older people often have to make a special effort to take regular exercise. Do you know any adults who go running, play squash, or go for long bike rides?

Rest and sleep

Your body cannot keep active for 24 hours a day. It needs time to **rest and recover**. The amount of **sleep** needed varies from person to person.

A new-born baby sleeps for between 16 and 18 hours a day. You probably have about 8 to 10 hours sleep a day. Generally, adults need less sleep than children, about 7 hours a day. Older people have about 7 hours at night, and often an hour or so during the day.

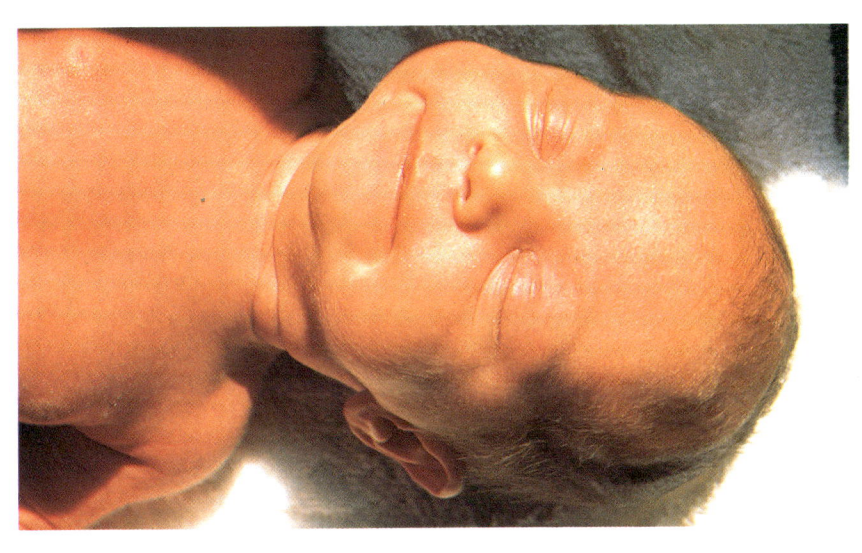

Babies need a lot of sleep because they grow quickly.

 You lose weight each night during sleep. Most people lose about 350 g.

Why do we sleep?

When you are asleep, your body rests, grows, and repairs itself. If you are ill, you usually need more sleep, in order to recover quickly. Your body never really switches off totally. Your brain rests although it is still active during sleep. Your muscles relax and your heartbeat slows down.

 Focus   exercise   heart   rest and recover   sleep

KEEPING HEALTHY

Germs

Germs are types of **microbes**. These are tiny living things that are too small to be seen without a microscope. Microbes (germs) include **viruses**, **bacteria**, and **fungi**. Some microbes cause you to be ill. The tiniest microbes are viruses. The next size up are bacteria, and the largest are fungi.

There are many different types of microbe that can cause you to be become ill.

- different viruses cause
  - colds
  - measles
  - mumps
- different bacteria cause
  - whooping cough
  - pneumonia
  - food poisoning
- different fungi cause
  - athlete's foot
  - ringworm

Colds and sneezes

Colds are caused by viruses. If your friend has a bad cold and sneezes, the cold viruses are thrown out into the air. You might breathe in some of them. They will quickly settle in your throat or in your nose, and begin to spread. The chances are that you will soon have a cold too.

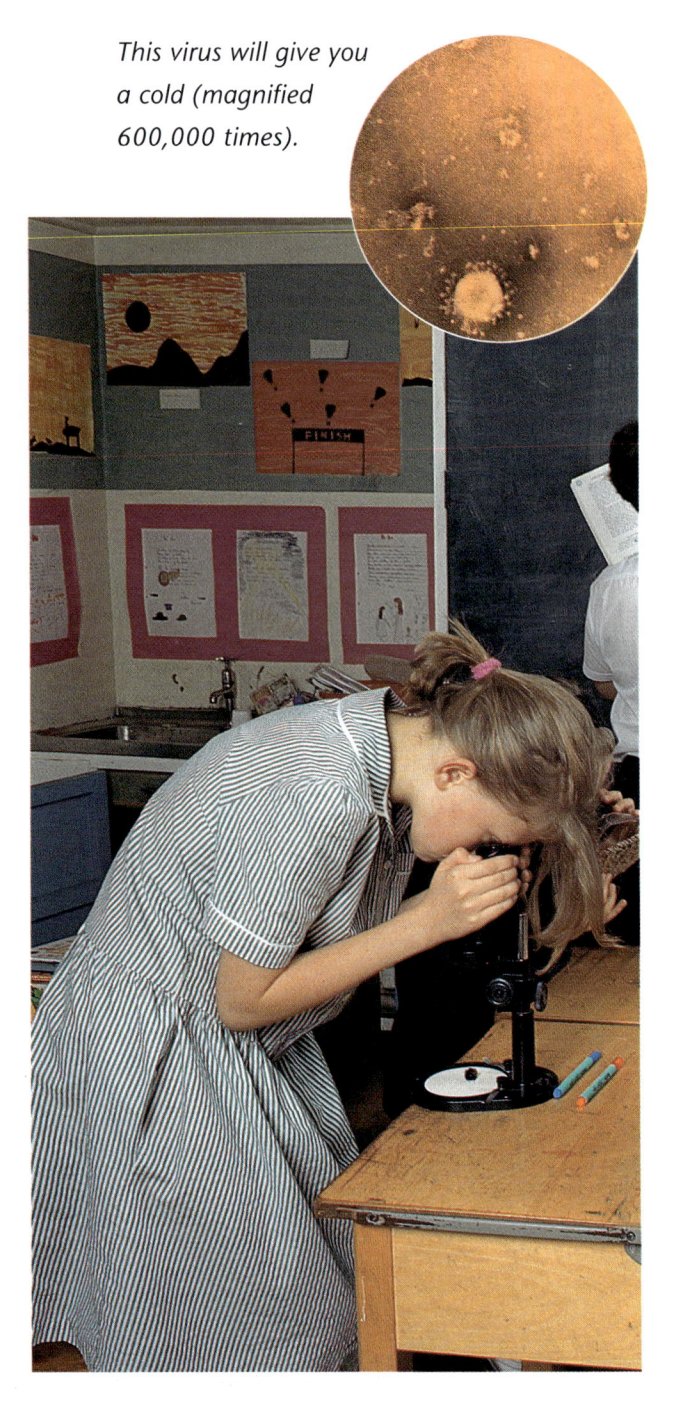

This virus will give you a cold (magnified 600,000 times).

School microscopes are not powerful enough to see microbes with.

The body's defence system

You already know that your **white blood cells** help your body to fight against microbes which cause illnesses. One kind of white cell surrounds microbes and destroys them.

Another kind of white blood cell makes substances called **antibodies**. Antibodies fight against germs and protect your body from illnesses. When the microbes have been destroyed some of the antibodies remain. They help to protect you in the future from the other microbes of the same type.

You have extra white blood cells in parts of your body called the lymph nodes. These cells also help in attacking harmful microbes.

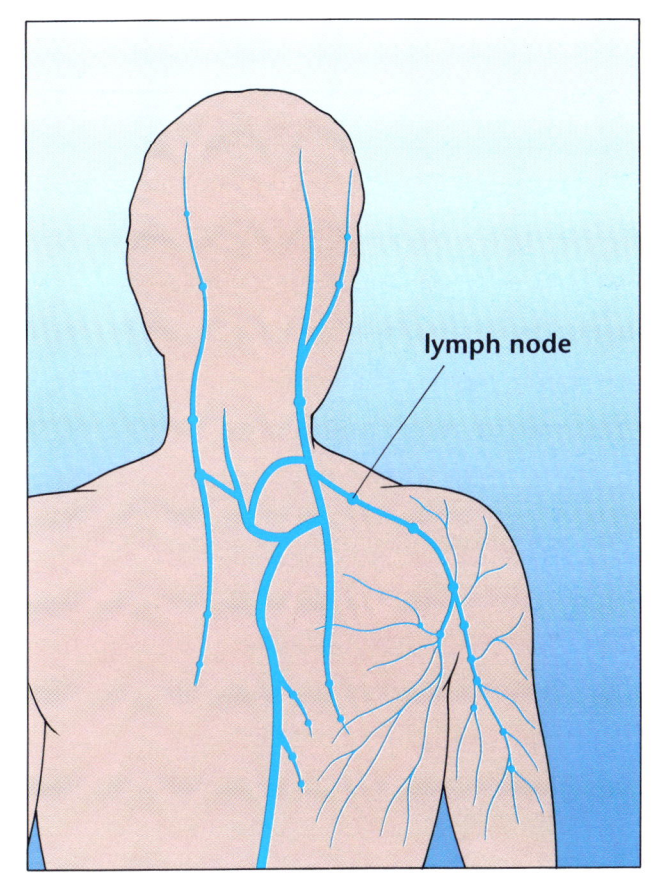

Your lymph nodes produce more white blood cells to fight 'germs'.

Becoming immune

You will probably have between eight and ten colds a year. As you grow older, your body will develop more antibodies and you should catch fewer colds. This means you become **immune** to certain types of microbes. If you are immune from certain microbes, your body is protected against them.

🍏 **Your body can make about 100,000 different antibodies to fight against different microbes.**

🍏 Focus

microbe

virus

bacterium

fungus

white blood cell

antibody

immune

39

● KEEPING HEALTHY

Medicines and drugs

However much care you take about eating a good diet, having regular exercise and looking after yourself, you will sometimes become ill.

You might need medicines

When you are ill you may need to take **medicines**. Some medicines are liquids you drink and some are pills you swallow. Other medicines could be ointments or creams to rub onto your body, and some could be injections.

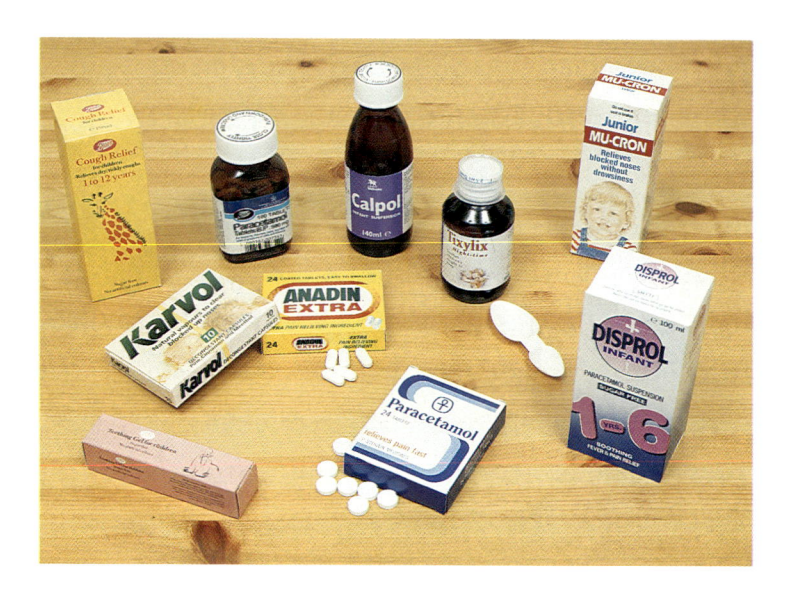

You should never touch any medicine without an adult knowing. It is very important to follow the instructions carefully.

Where do you get medicines?

If you visit the doctor and you need medicine, you will be given a **prescription**. A prescription gives details of the amount of a particular medicine you need. You hand the prescription to a person in the chemist's shop, and they will make the medicine ready for you. The label on the medicine container will tell you exactly what the medicine is called. It also says how much you need to take and how often.

All medicines are drugs

Drugs are important in relieving or curing illnesses. However, they are dangerous if misused. When drugs are used in a way for which they are not intended, people can become **addicted**. **Addiction** to drugs means that the user cannot stop themselves from taking the drug every day.

40

Smoking

You know that smoking causes lung cancer and that lung cancer usually leads to death. Yet many people still smoke. Smokers are addicted to a drug inside the tobacco called nicotine. Nicotine affects the heart, the blood system, and the nervous system.

Drinking

Alcohol can be an addictive drug. Many adults enjoy a glass of wine or beer from time to time. Drinking in sensible amounts does no harm at all. However, some people become addicted to alcohol. They find it impossible to go through a day without having large quantities of alcoholic drink. Alcohol can cause diseases of the liver, kidneys, and bloodstream.

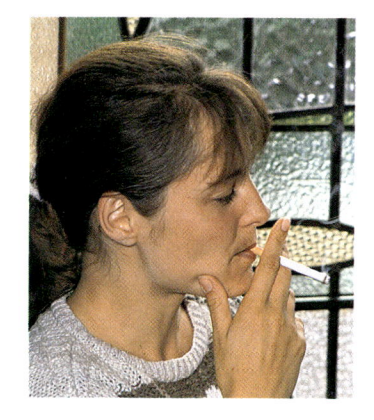

It is easy to become addicted to nicotine, but hard to break the addiction.

'Designer drugs'

A dangerous development in the misuse of drugs is the appearance of so-called 'designer drugs'. These can be bought at some night clubs and parties, often by teenagers. These young people do not realize that taking drugs *may* lead to an early death.

Solvent abuse

Many medicines (and some other materials) have to be dissolved in a liquid before they are used. There are many kinds of these special liquids. They are called solvents. These solvents are meant to be swallowed together with the medicines. Some solvents evaporate very easily and people become addicted to the vapour. This is solvent abuse.

🍎 **All medicines are drugs but not all drugs are medicines.**

🍎 **Focus**   medicine   prescription   drug   addicted   addiction

GENETICS

What you look like

Next time you see your friends or your family, look closely at them. In what ways are they the same as you, and in what ways they are different from you?

Unless you have an identical twin, no-one looks exactly like you. But there will be similarities between you and the rest of your family.

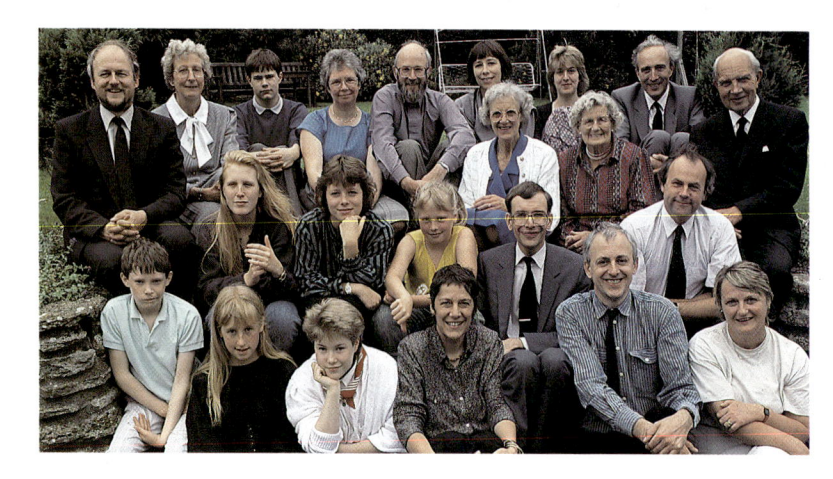

In what ways are you like the rest of your family?

Twins

You might be a twin or you might know twins in your school or neighbourhood. Twins who are alike are called **identical twins**. If they are unlike or of different sexes, they are called **fraternal twins**.

Identical twins have eyes and hair the same colour and even eyebrows of the same shape. Friends and teachers can find it difficult to tell identical twins apart. Sometimes even the fingerprints of identical twins are almost the same.

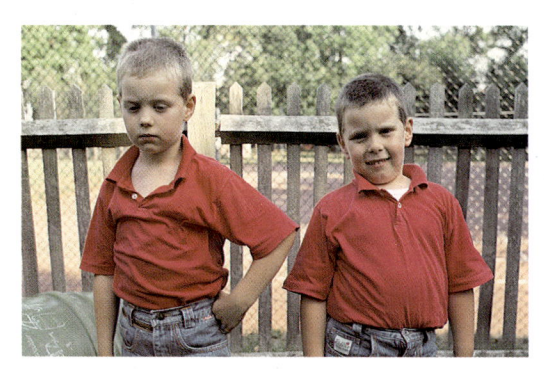

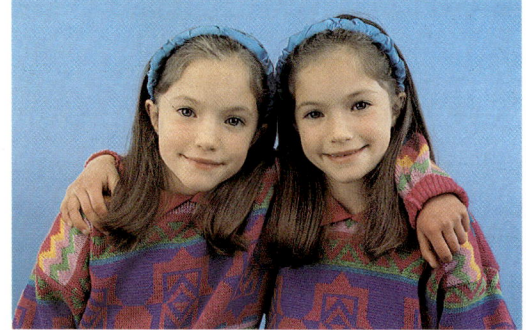

It is much easier to tell the difference between fraternal twins than identical twins!

Why do you look like your parents?

You know that you began life as a **single cell**. The centre of the cell is called the **nucleus**. Inside this nucleus were a group of fine twisted threads called **chromosomes**. Chromosomes contain thousands of **instructions** passed on from your mother and father. Your chromosomes are different from everyone else's and they make you a unique individual. The thousands of instructions, which are like the plans for the growth of your body, are called **genes**.

How do genes work?

When you were developing as a baby inside your mother's womb, your genes were busy. Every growing cell received an exact copy of all of your chromosomes and their genes. These genes controlled how each cell developed.

As you have genes from both your father and mother, you inherit **characteristics** from them both (red hair, curly hair, blue eyes...). Characteristics are also passed on from generation to generation. You will probably share some characteristics with your grandparent's grandparents!

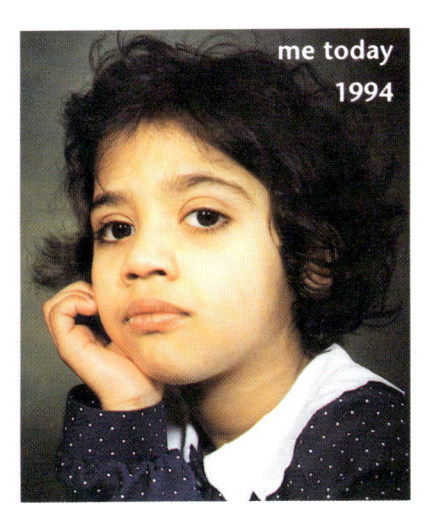

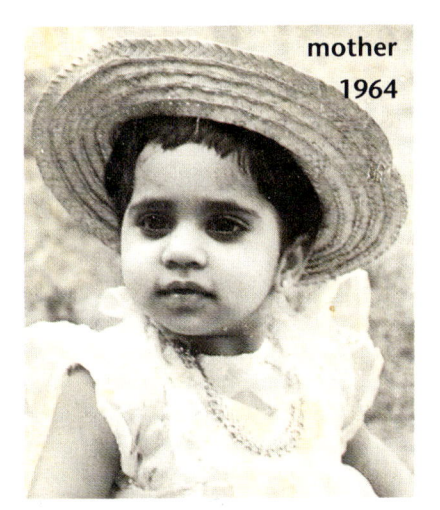

Focus

identical twin
fraternal twin
single cell
nucleus
chromosome
instruction
gene
characteristic

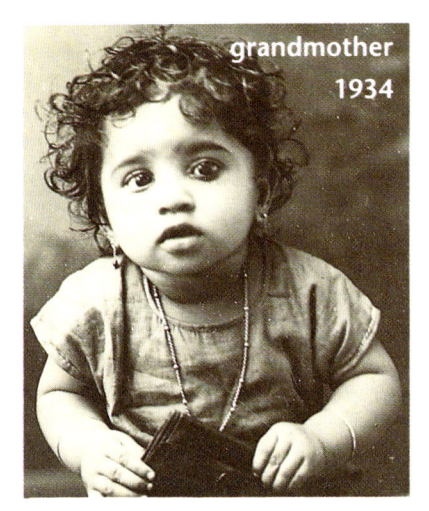

Characteristics can be passed on through many different generations.

GENETICS

It runs in the family

How did you come to be a boy?
Why did you turn out to be a girl?
The answer to these questions can be found in chromosomes.

Chromosomes in cells

Every single **cell** in an adult's body has 46 **chromosomes**, apart from the sex cells. The **sex cells** are the **sperm cells** of the male and the **egg cells** of the female. The sperm cells and the egg cells contain 23 chromosomes each. When these join together to make the very first cell of a new baby, they make up the full number of 46 chromosomes.

Boy or girl?

There is one sex characteristic out of the 23 chromosomes in both the egg and the sperm.
The sex chromosomes are called 'X' and 'Y'. All eggs have an 'X' chromosome.
Half of a man's sperms have 'Y' and half have 'X' chromosomes,
If a sperm with a 'Y' chromosome joins the egg, the baby will be a boy (Y *and* X).
If a sperm with an 'X' chromosome joins the egg, the baby will be a girl (X *and* X).

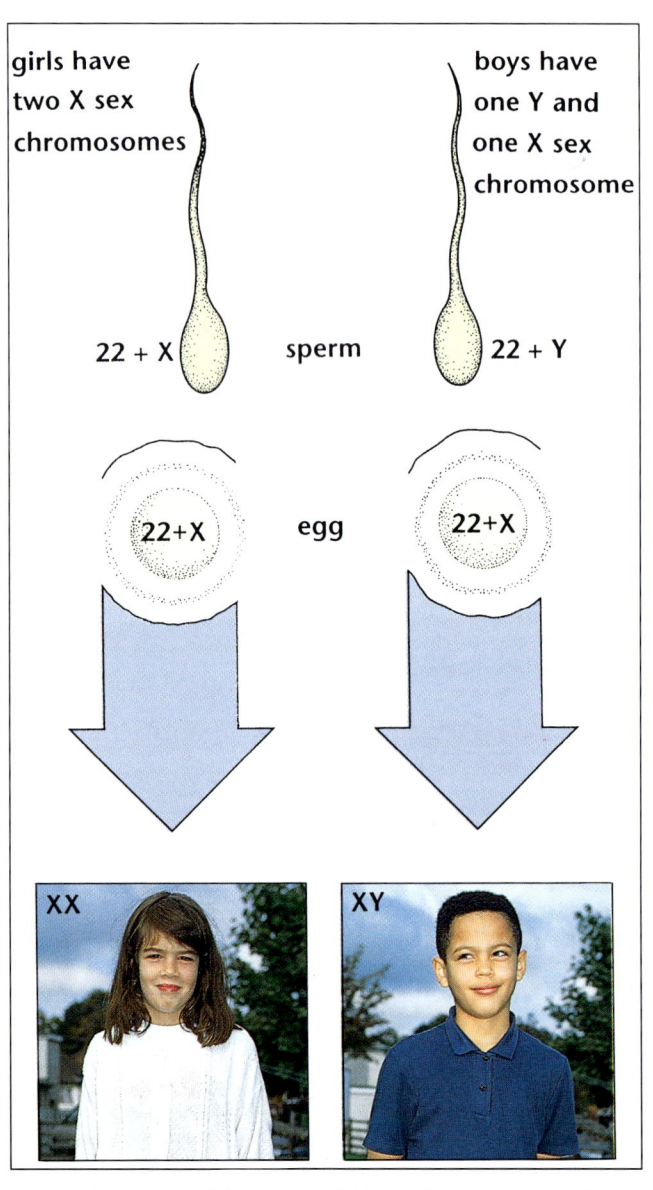

girls have two X sex chromosomes

boys have one Y and one X sex chromosome

sperm: 22 + X | 22 + Y

egg: 22+X | 22+X

XX | XY

Boys have one 'Y' and one 'X' sex chromosome. Girls have two 'X' sex chromosomes.

44

Down's syndrome

If a developing baby gets an extra chromosome from one or both parents, this can cause a problem. **Down's syndrome** is when the baby has three of a particular chromosome instead of the normal two. This means the baby has 47 chromosomes instead of 46. This tiny difference affects the mental and physical development of the individual throughout its life.

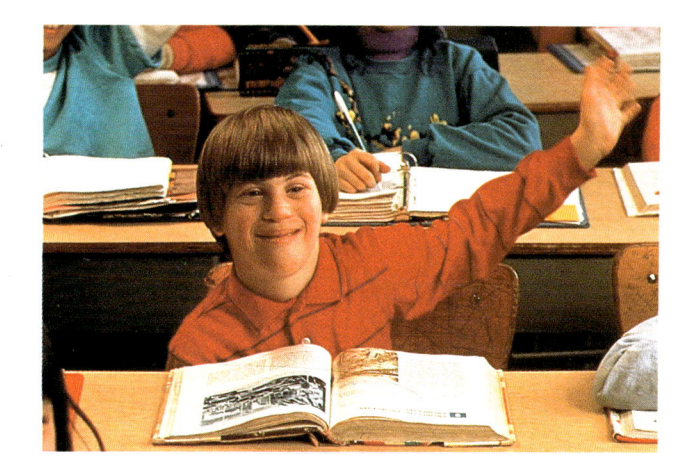

People with Down's syndrome have an extra chromosome.

How is a gene made up?

A chromosome is made up of a number of smaller sections called genes. A gene is a series of chemicals. Every gene is made up of a series of chemicals, all joined together like a twisted ladder. The order of the chemicals varies in each gene. These chemicals make up rungs of the twisted ladder, Each gene is an instruction. A particular sequence of rungs gives the instructions for a characteristic, such as hair colour.

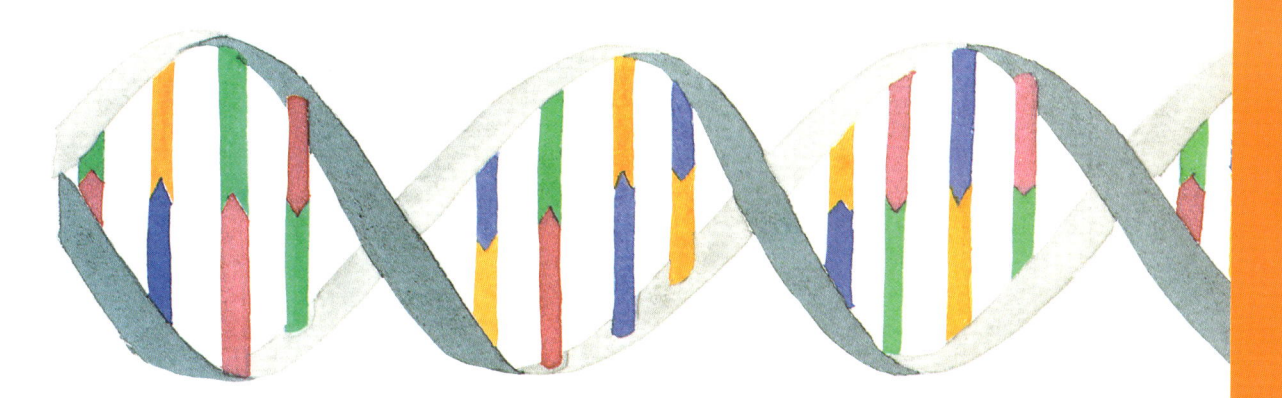

The 'twisted' ladder containing instructions for genes is known as a DNA molecule.

Focus   cell   chromosome   sex cell   sperm cell   egg cell   Down's syndrome

45

GROWING UP

Growing up, growing older

You started life smaller than a pin head. Everyone began life as just one tiny cell. This one cell was made during a time called **fertilization**. Fertilization happens when a **sperm** from a man's body enters an **egg** in a woman's body.

After a few hours, the single cell divides into two. Over the next eight to nine months, the number of cells increases and a **baby** grows inside the woman's womb for about 38 weeks.

A baby growing

When you were a baby, you grew very quickly. You were fed regularly and your cells continually increased in number. When you were just one year old, you were about four times your birth weight.

Childhood

Throughout childhood you continue growing. When girls are about seven years old and boys are about nine years old, they are about three-quarters of their adult height.

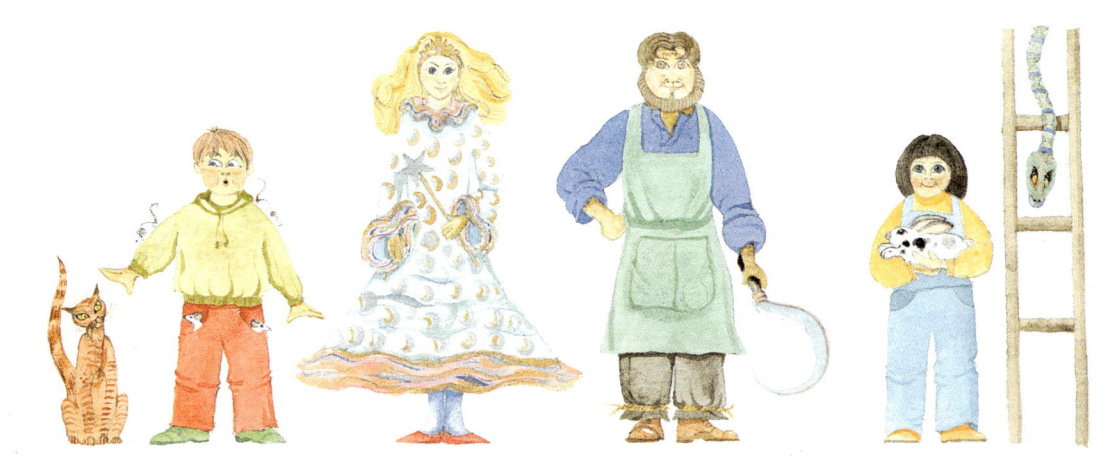

You reach about three-quarters of your adult height between the ages of 7 and 9.

Adolescence

Adolescence comes between childhood and adulthood. During this time changes take place in your body. This stage of development is called **puberty**. Some of these changes are:

boys start puberty at about 13 years:
- hair begins to grow on the face and body
- muscle weight develops
- height may increase
- shoulders and chest become broader
- the voice gets deeper
- sex organs enlarge
- interest begins in the opposite sex

girls start puberty at about 11 years:
- breasts start to develop
- voice gets a little lower
- hips become broader
- body hair starts to grow
- height may increase
- the ability to give birth becomes possible
- interest begins in the opposite sex

Adulthood

The stage between adolescence and adulthood marks the end of your physical growing. Your amazing body machine is complete when you become an adult. Take a look at the adults you know. See how their lives are different from yours.

When life ends

Every living thing has to die. Someone could die because of an illness or accident. As people get older, and into old age, their body cells wear out. They are unable to fight against illness and disease like a younger person.

When a friend or relative dies it is a sad time for everyone. Death is the last stage of the human **life cycle**.

● In 1815, the average life span of a European adult was about 39 years. Today it is 75 years.

● **Focus**   fertilization   sperm   egg   baby   puberty   life cycle

Index

*Note: the main reference for multiple entries is given in **bold** print.*

addiction   40
adulthood   47
anorexia nervosa   33
antibodies   39
anus   12
arms   2
arteries   17

bacteria   29, **38**
bladder   6, **13**
blood   7, 8, **14**, 15, 23, 29, 36,39
bloodstream   **10**, 13, 14
bones   **20**, 21
brain   6, **18**, 19, 24, 25, 26, 27, 37
breathing   8

capillaries   17
carbon dioxide   8
cells   **4**, 5, 6, 10, 13, 14, 22, 24, 29, 44, 46, 47
chromosomes   **43**, 44

defence system   14, **39**
diet   30
digestion   7, **10**, 13
digestive system   10, **11**, 23
Down's syndrome   45
drugs   40

ears   6, **25**
elbow   21
energy   10
eyes   3, 6, **24**

exercise   36

faeces   12
famine   32
fertilisation   46
food   **10**, 12, 30, 32, 33, 35
fungi   38

genes   43
germs   34, 35, **38**

haemoglobin   14
haemophilia   15
hair   3
head   2
hearing   24, **25**
heart   6, 7, **16**, 36
heart disease   33
hygiene   35

immunity   39
intestines   6, **11**, 12

joints   21

kidneys   6, **13**, 17

legs   2
life cycle   47
life expectancy   33
lungs   6, 7, **8**, 9,16, 26
lung cancer   9
lymph nodes   39

malnutrition   32
medicines   40

microbes   38
muscles   2, 7, **22**, 23, 36

nerves   **18**, 26, 28
nervous system   18
nucleus   **5**, 43
nutrients   **10**, 30, 31

obesity   33
oesophagus   11
optic nerve   24
organs   6
oxygen   **8**, 9, 14, 16

personal hygiene   34
plasma   14
puberty   47
pupil   24

rectum   12
reflex action   19
retina   24

salmonella   35
senses   **24**, 26, 28
sex cells   44
sight   24
skeleton   2, **20**, 23
skin   2, 3, **28**, 29
skull   18
sleep   37
smell   **26**, 27
smoking   9, **41**
sperm   46
spinal cord   **18**, 20
spine   20

stomach   7, **10**, 11
sweat   29

taste   26, **27**
teeth   34
tongue   27
touch   28
trunk   2
twins   42

urine   13

veins   17
viruses   38

waste   3, 5, **12**, 13, 31
wind pipe   11

Oxford University Press, Walton Street, Oxford OX2 6DP

*Oxford   New York   Toronto
Delhi   Bombay   Calcutta   Madras   Karachi
Kuala Lumpur   Singapore   Hong Kong   Tokyo
Nairobi   Dar es Salaam   Cape Town
Melbourne   Auckland   Madrid*

and associated companies in
Berlin   Ibadan

Oxford is a trademark of the Oxford University Press

© Steve Blackman 1994

First published 1994

ISBN 0 19 918323 6

A CIP record for this book is available from the British Library.

All rights reserved. No part of this publication may be reproduced, stored in a retrieval system, or transmitted, in any form or by any means, without the prior permission in writing of Oxford University Press. Within the UK, exceptions are allowed in respect of any fair dealing for the purpose of research or private study, or criticism or review, as permitted under the Copyright, Designs and Patents Act, 1988, or in the case of reprographic reproduction in accordance with the terms of licences issued by the Copyright Licensing Agency. Enquiries concerning reproduction outside those terms and in other countries should be sent to the Rights Department, Oxford University Press, at the address above.

Acknowledgements

The publisher wishes to thank the following for supplying photographs:

Allsport p 29; Sally & Richard Greenhill pp 10, 33 (bottom), 42 (top & bottom left); L Menon p 43 (all); Science Photo Library p 45, /M Kage p 4, /B Iverson p 4, /M Walker p 4, /P Motta p 4, /Moredun Animal Health Ltd p 5, /J Stevenson p 9 (all), /A Syred p 14, /P Plailly p 15, /M Kage p 20, /J Stevenson p 21 (all), /Moredun Animal Health Ltd p 35 (left), /J Wachter p 36 (bottom left), /J Stevenson p 37, /J Selby p 38, /Dr S Patterson p 38 (inset), /D Lovegrove p 41; Stills /T Hormbak p 32.

Additional photography by Chris Honeywell.

Cover photograph by Pictor International.

Special thanks to East Oxford First School.

The illustrations are by:

Nicky Cooney and Oxford Illustrators.

Printed in France by Pollina, 85400 Luçon - n° 65428 - A